THE OWNER'S MANUAL TO THE VOICE

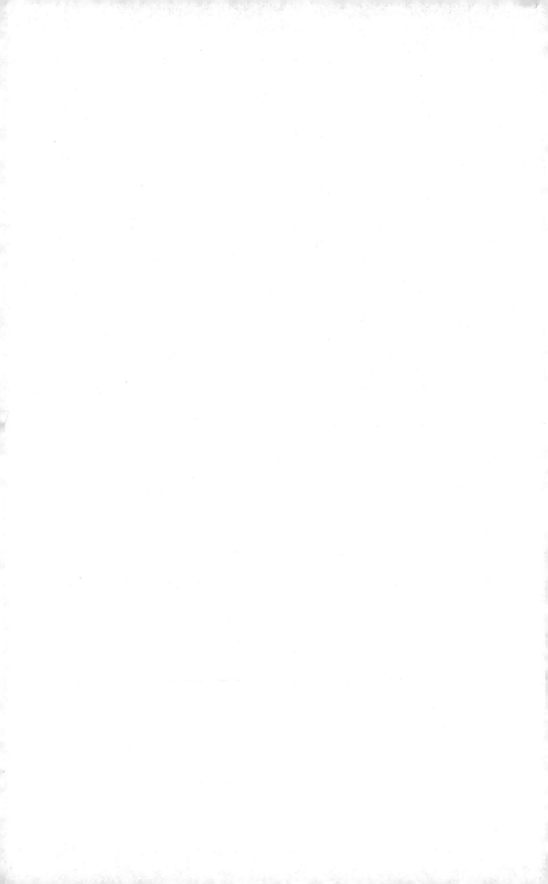

The Owner's Manual to the Voice

A GUIDE FOR SINGERS AND OTHER
PROFESSIONAL VOICE USERS

Rachael Gates, D.M.A.

L. Arick Forrest, M.D.

Kerrie Obert, M.A., C.C.C/S.L.P.

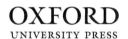

OXFORD
UNIVERSITY PRESS

Oxford University Press is a department of the University of Oxford.
It furthers the University's objective of excellence in research, scholarship,
and education by publishing worldwide.

Oxford   New York
Auckland   Cape Town   Dar es Salaam   Hong Kong   Karachi
Kuala Lumpur   Madrid   Melbourne   Mexico City   Nairobi
New Delhi   Shanghai   Taipei   Toronto

With offices in
Argentina   Austria   Brazil   Chile   Czech Republic   France   Greece
Guatemala   Hungary   Italy   Japan   Poland   Portugal   Singapore
South Korea   Switzerland   Thailand   Turkey   Ukraine   Vietnam

Oxford is a registered trademark of Oxford University Press in the UK and certain other
countries.

Published in the United States of America by
Oxford University Press
198 Madison Avenue, New York, NY 10016

Library of Congress Cataloging-in-Publication Data
Gates, Rachael.
The owner's manual to the voice : a guide for singers and other professional voice users/
Rachael Gates, Arick Forrest, Kerrie Obert.
p. cm.
Includes bibliographical references and index.
ISBN 978–0–19–996466–6 (alk. paper)—ISBN 978–0–19–996468–0 (alk. paper)   1. Voice—Care and
hygiene   2. Voice culture.   3. Voice—Physiological aspects.   I. Forrest, Arick.   II. Obert,
Kerrie.   III. Title.
MT821.G38 2013
783'.043—dc23
2012041874

1 3 5 7 9 8 6 4 2
Printed in the United States of America
on acid-free paper

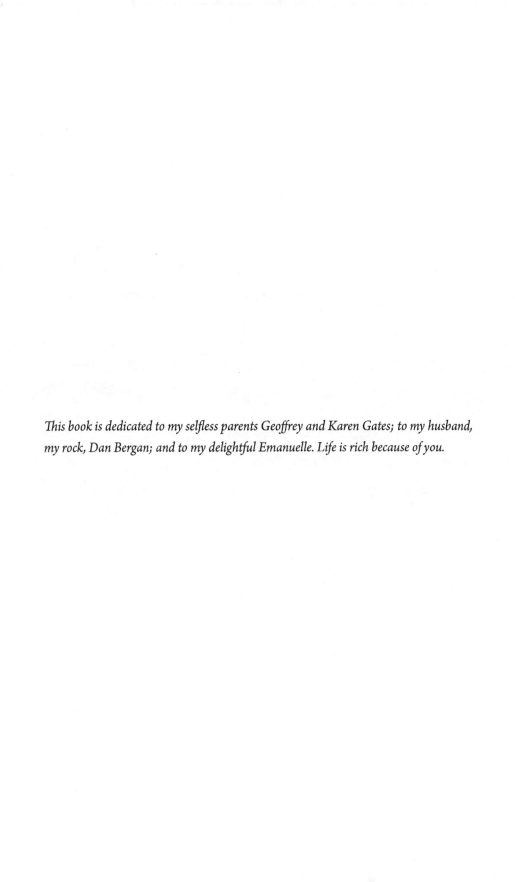

This book is dedicated to my selfless parents Geoffrey and Karen Gates; to my husband, my rock, Dan Bergan; and to my delightful Emanuelle. Life is rich because of you.

Contents

Figures, Tables, and Video Clips

TABLES

▶ VIDEO CLIPS

Acknowledgments

WE ARE SO pleased that our wonderful editor (and singer), Suzanne Ryan, gave us her "vibrant green light to move forward." We are also appreciative for the excellent communications and expertise of OUP editor Norman Hirschy, assistant editor Adam Cohen, contract manager Richard Kelaher, copyeditor Danielle Michaely, and Molly Morrison of Newgen North America.

Thank you.

We are grateful for all the colleagues at the Voice & Swallowing Disorders Clinic at the Ohio State University Wexner Medical Center who helped in this process. We specifically thank Michelle Toth, MA, CCC/SLP; Jennifer Thompson, MA, CCC/SLP; Eugene Chio, MD; and Brad deSilva, MD, for helping to gather pathology images. We are indebted to Joy Landis of Michigan State University for her tireless attention and technical expertise in helping to prepare all of the images used in this book. We are grateful for the many patients who allowed the use of their pathology images and for all of the patients and students who continue to inspire.

I, Rachael Gates, have been careful to give credit when using words from others, but please let me know if I have left out credit where it is due.

I will forever sing the praises of all the friends and colleagues who were generous with their time and talents in creating this book, particularly:

Greg Upton, my wonderful first voice teacher, who said, "You're going to sing, not go into medicine,"

Michael D. Trudeau, for enabling my independent study,

Robin Rice, for bringing out the best in my voice and teaching me how to teach,

Loretta Robinson, for being an attentive advisor,

Karen Peeler, for the inspiring pedagogy class,

Don Penner and Rose and Tali Snyder, for technical help and extra support,

Johari Parnell, for allowing me to stand by her during her phonosurgery,

Johannes Müller Stosch, for the idea to write this in the first place,

Peggy Crum, Jan Fonarow, Anna Gates, Ken Gross, Molly Guerin, Chi and Kristin Huang, Walter and Nancy Hull, Esther Park, and Katherine Verdolini—all experts in their fields and generous with their knowledge,

Adam Bohman and Stephen Crump of KayPENTAX, for video clips and clinical instrument details,

Quoc Le, for excellent prosection photos,

Rick Meurs, for prompt and efficient work on illustrations,

Rebecca Pratt and Anthony Paganini, for readily answering questions and inviting me to frequent the MSU Gross Anatomy Lab,

The men and women who generously donated their bodies after death to the MSU Division of Human Anatomy's Willed Body Program,

Sherrill Milnes, inspiring colleague, for reading and enjoying this text,

Rachel Webster, for expert proofing and amazing encouragement,

Carol and Don Stallard, Steve and Laning Thompson, Roseanna Irwin, Pamela Jordan Schiffer, Judy Palac, Ashley Ahlin, Bay Warren, and Karen Behm, for generous support,

My supportive family—Rita O'Leary Keener, Kathleen and John Berglund, David Keener, Bill and Colleen Keener, Tom O'Leary, Meri Lee Perkins, David and Jane Gates,

and

The Bergan Family, loving in-laws, for their valuable advice.

About the Authors

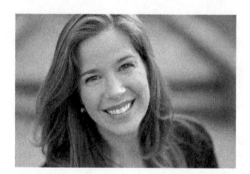

Soprano, Opera Director, and Singing Health Specialist, Dr. Rachael Gates has sung in Germany, Italy, Russia, and throughout the United States. She has taught at Northwestern University, The Hartt School of Music, and has guest-directed operas for Yale University. She teaches vocal health at Michigan State University where she is a member of the MSU Musician's Wellness Team. She holds degrees from Carnegie Mellon University, Cincinnati College–Conservatory of Music, and The Ohio State University where she received her Doctorate of Musical Arts.

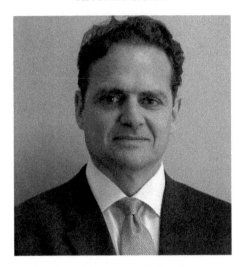

Dr. L. Arick Forrest is the Vice Chairman of the Department of Otolaryngology, Residency Program Director, and serves as the Director of The Ohio State University Voice and Swallowing Disorders Clinic. He has been involved in treating the professional voice since completing his laryngology fellowship at Vanderbilt University under Robert H. Ossoff, DMD, MD, in 1993.

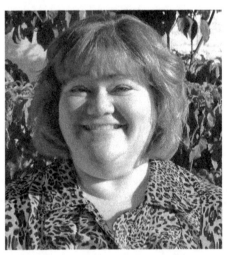

Kerrie Beechler Obert, MA-CCC/SLP, is a clinical voice pathologist at The Ohio State University Voice and Swallowing Disorders Clinic in Columbus, Ohio. A graduate of Mars Hill College (NC) and The Ohio State University, Ms. Obert's research interests are geared toward the professional voice community. Ms. Obert holds degrees in speech pathology and music and she has extensive performance training in a variety of styles and techniques. She has published articles on voice quality and is co-author of an anatomy textbook, *Geography of the Voice: Anatomy of an Adam's Apple*, with Steven R. Chicurel, DMA, as well as two course workbooks, *Estill Voice Training Level One: Compulsory Figures for Voice Control and Estill Voice Training Level Two: Figure Combinations for Six Voice Qualities*.

How to Use This Book

THIS BOOK IS written primarily for singers but is also relevant to all types of professional voice users and medical professionals as well. The information presented in each chapter builds from vocabulary presented in previous chapters. For this reason, you may find it helpful to read this book front to back. However, if you already have a basic understanding of vocal anatomy, function, and terminology, this text also serves as a quick and useful reference with easily accessible answers to your questions or concerns. The use of "he" and "she" throughout the text reflects the roles and sexes of the authors. Therefore, when referring to a singer, clinician, or speech-language pathologist, "she" is used, and when a physician or an anesthesiologist is mentioned, "he" is used. This choice is meant to simplify and not to promote stereotypes. To be applicable to medical professionals and to countries outside the United States, anatomical structures are measured using the metric system and in many instances the USA/Imperial System as well. Additional bits of information on topics can be found in boxes throughout each chapter and are marked either "Anecdote," "Note," or "Warning." New vocabulary is in bold and definitions can be found in the extensive alphabetized glossary at the back of the book. Pronunciations are given for words that may be difficult to pronounce. Would you like to look up a medicine's potential to affect the voice? Search the index by the medicine's classification or generic name to locate more information in the text. Some common brand names are indexed as well. Commercially manufactured medicines and products are capitalized and followed with their trademark symbol when listed in this book (e.g. Alka-Seltzer®). No commercial company participated in the writing of this book and none of the companies are responsible for the accuracy of the information regarding their products listed here. The information presented in this book is for self-edification and not a substitute for professional care.

About the Companion Website

ALL VIDEO FOOTAGE mentioned in this book and full-color versions of the images included in this text are available and further discussed on the following website:

www.oup.com/us/theownersmanualtothevoice

You may access this companion website by typing in username Music3 and password Book3234.

THE OWNER'S MANUAL TO THE VOICE

I

Introduction

AS SINGERS, WE talk about our voice as an intangible phenomenon and take for granted its physiological functions. But what happens when something goes wrong? What do we do when something feels wrong? To whom can we turn and in whom can we trust? We go on voice rest and blame it on stress, a sore throat, a cold, the weather, being out of shape, being physically tired, oversinging, and so forth. How could we have prevented "it" and ensure "it" won't happen again?

We trust our voice teachers' empathetic ears and long history of experience. We go to the doctor or drug store for medications. But what is going on with our instrument? How can we be sure that the measures we decide to take are the best ones?

As singers, we are in tune with our voices and use them in an athletically vigorous and intricately detailed way. With discipline and good technique, our instruments appear refreshingly healthy and perhaps even muscularly toned. Because of this, a singer with a complaint may be dismissed as healthy by **physicians** who rarely care for singers and are accustomed to seeing severe vocal disorders and maladies. Subtle changes in the **vocal folds** are often overlooked or not perceived, even by ear, nose, and throat specialists. By the singer's standards, however, the voice is functioning poorly. The singer's livelihood relies on being able to communicate specifically with the physician about the condition of the instrument. This manual enables singers to understand their instrument and provides an overview of possible medical conditions that may occur in an approachable way.

2

Your Instrument at a Glance

IN THIS CHAPTER we will take a tour of some basic anatomy involved in voice production. We are going to guide you through locating this anatomy on your own body
and help you visualize what you cannot see. The figures in this chapter are not ordered
sequentially as they are discussed in the text. Rather, they have been grouped together
to create an easy reference point and, more importantly, to help you gain a better 3-D
understanding of the anatomy discussed in this book. Please turn back to these figures as
needed to clarify anatomical references as they're mentioned throughout the text.

To virtually navigate the anatomy discussed in this chapter, we will occasionally employ
directional terms used by medical professionals. Please refer to Figure 2 as a reference
when you are confused by this terminology.

2.1 WHERE IS IT?

Put your fingers on the front of your neck. Can you feel a bump? Your instrument lies
directly behind that bump. The bump is made of cartilage and, like an instrument case, is
designed to protect the two tiny bands of vibrating **tissue** we call vocal folds. The bump
tends to stick out more distinctly on men than on women and is commonly referred to as
an Adam's apple. This protrusion at the front of the neck is the prominent feature of the
thyroid cartilage. Now feel for a steep little dip at the top of the bump called the **thyroid
notch**. Your vocal folds attach just behind and below that thyroid notch.

You may have difficulty when first trying to find the thyroid cartilage. On some female
necks, another cartilage protrudes more obviously than the thyroid. This cartilage is the
cricoid, which actually sits just below the thyroid cartilage. What may further confuse

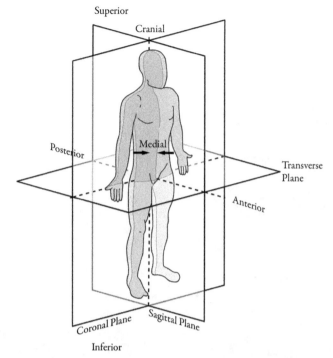

FIGURE 2 Anatomical Planes and Directions

Superior (above), inferior (below), anterior (in front of, toward the front), posterior (behind, toward the back), medial (toward the middle), cranial (toward the head), coronal (divides an object vertically front to back), **sagittal** (divides an object vertically/longitudinally side to side), transverse (divides an object horizontally into top and bottom). Not labeled: median (the middle, center of an object), lateral (pertaining to the side), superficial (near the surface, opposite of deep).

you is that the cricoid cartilage dips slightly in the front and you may mistake this dip to be the thyroid notch. To avoid mistaking the two and to further understand the structure of your instrument, let's do a little more bodymapping.

2.2 BODYMAPPING

Drag a finger down along the underneath of your chin until you reach the top of the neck. (See Figures 2.2a and 2.2b.) Gently massage until you locate the V-like dip of the thyroid notch. If you place the pad of your index finger in the dip, the tip of your fingernail will touch a small ridge of bone just above called the **hyoid**. The hyoid bone is one of two free-floating bones in the body and is the body's only bone that has no relationship to another bone! It is a horseshoe-shaped bone, closed at the front of the neck and open toward the back of the neck, and sits suspended in soft tissues under the base of the tongue. It measures about 3.3 to 3.5 cm (1.35 inches) from front to back and 4 cm (1.57 inches) from tip to tip at the opening of the "U."[1] From it hang the rest of the cartilages, via **membranes** and **ligaments**, which make up your voice box or **larynx**.

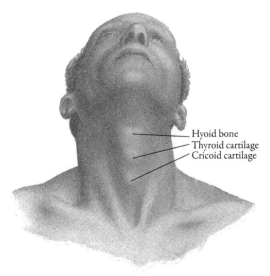

FIGURE 2.2a Bodymapping, Anterior View of Neck

Hyoid bone
Thyroid cartilage
Cricoid cartilage

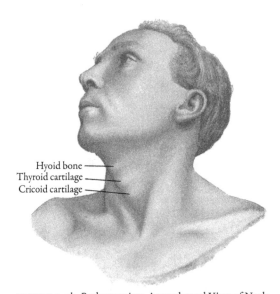

Hyoid bone
Thyroid cartilage
Cricoid cartilage

FIGURE 2.2b Bodymapping, Anterolateral View of Neck

Note: Other than the hyoid, the knee cap or patella is the only free-floating bone in the body. Neither attaches to another bone but instead is suspended by muscles, **tendons**, or ligaments. Unlike the hyoid, which has no relationship to another bone whatsoever, the patella does glide in a groove on the femur bone just behind it.

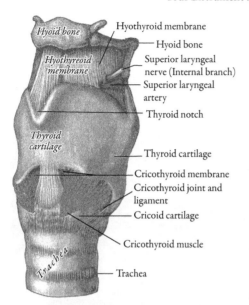

Hyoid bone

Hyothyreoid
membrane

Thyroid
cartilage

Trachea

Hyothyroid membrane
Hyoid bone
Superior laryngeal
nerve (Internal branch)
Superior laryngeal
artery
Thyroid notch

Thyroid cartilage

Cricothyroid membrane
Cricothyroid joint and
ligament
Cricoid cartilage

Cricothyroid muscle

Trachea

FIGURE 2.2c Anterolateral View of Larynx

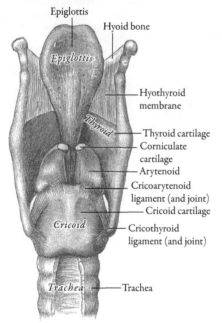

Epiglottis

Hyoid bone

Epiglottis

Thyroid

Cricoid

Trachea

Hyothyroid
membrane

Thyroid cartilage
Corniculate
cartilage
Arytenoid
Cricoarytenoid
ligament (and joint)
Cricoid cartilage
Cricothyroid
ligament (and joint)

Trachea

FIGURE 2.2d Posterior View of Larynx

Note: Medical literature uses the word "thyroid" alone to mean the thyroid gland. The thyroid gland is separate from the cartilage and not discussed in this text. You will find that we consistently use the word "thyroid" in conjunction with the word "cartilage" in this text, because we are always referring specifically to the cartilage and not to the thyroid gland.

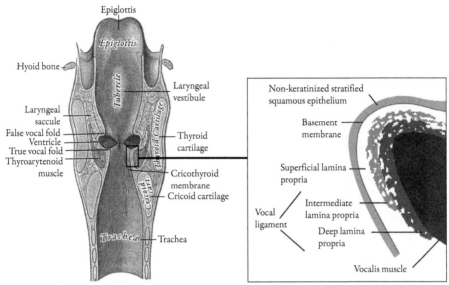

FIGURE 2.2e Posterior View of Larynx, Coronal Cut: general view (left) and detail (right)
Mucosal linings and muscle added. Left: The box outlining the right vocal fold marks the section enlarged in the detail. Right: Illustrated close-up of the right vocal fold coronal cut depicted in general view. The vocal fold's layers are simplified for clarity. Note that the vocalis muscle is labeled rather than the thyroarytenoid because the thyromuscularis band that runs lateral to the vocalis is not close enough to the vibrating edge to show here.

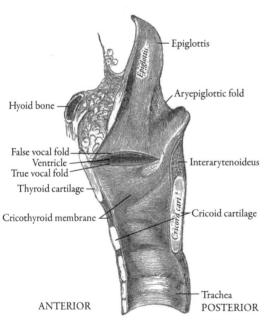

FIGURE 2.2f Sagittal Cut of Larynx and Upper Trachea
Mucosal linings and muscle added.

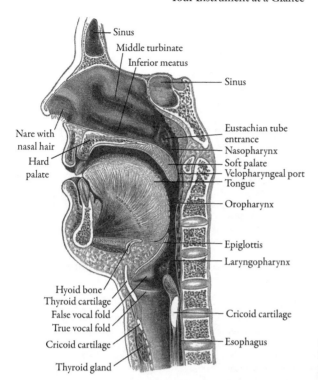

Sinus
Middle turbinate
Inferior meatus
Sinus
Nare with nasal hair
Eustachian tube entrance
Nasopharynx
Hard palate
Soft palate
Velopharyngeal port
Tongue
Oropharynx
Epiglottis
Laryngopharynx
Hyoid bone
Thyroid cartilage
False vocal fold
True vocal fold
Cricoid cartilage
Cricoid cartilage
Esophagus
Thyroid gland

FIGURE 2.2g Sagittal Cut of Nose, Mouth, Pharynx, and Larynx

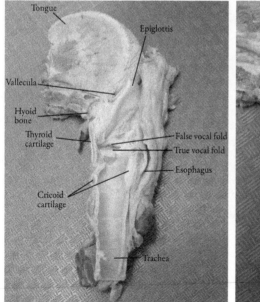
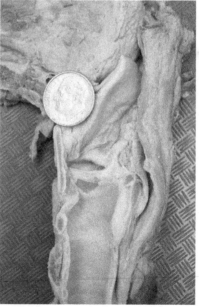

Tongue
Epiglottis
Vallecula
Hyoid bone
Thyroid cartilage
False vocal fold
True vocal fold
Esophagus
Cricoid cartilage
Trachea

FIGURE 2.2h Sagittal Cut of Tongue and Larynx: general view (A) and detail (B)
A: Cadaver **prosection**. B: Cadaver prosection shows laryngeal anatomy relative to a dime.

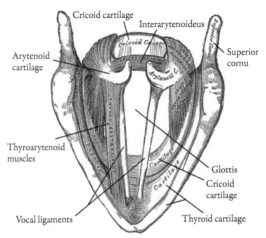

FIGURE 2.2i Larynx from Above
Illustration depicts an oral endoscope's view of vocal folds without mucosal linings. The two separate bands of muscle that make up the thyroarytenoids are not easy to distinguish here. The hyoid bone is not pictured.

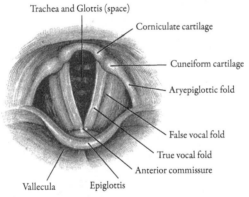

FIGURE 2.2j Larynx from Above (with mucosal linings)
Illustration depicts an oral endoscope's view of the vocal folds. The entrance to the esophagus is not labeled here, but it is the horizontal line at the top of the picture, just posterior to the folds. Refer to Figure 5.10 for further clarification.

With your finger still at the thyroid notch, trace down below the dip to grasp the size of this topmost and largest of the **laryngeal** cartilages called the thyroid cartilage. It is more than just a bump (a.k.a. laryngeal prominence). Feel how the thyroid cartilage

> Thyroid literally means "shield" in Greek. The thyroid cartilage is shaped like a shield and acts like a shield for the vocal folds.

---

[1] K. W. P. Miller, P. L. Walker, and R. L. O'Halloran, "Age and Sex-Related Variation in Hyoid Bone Morphology," *Journal of Forensic Science* 43, no. 6 (1998): 1138–1143.

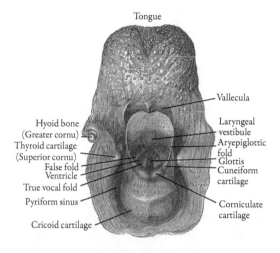

Tongue

Vallecula

Hyoid bone
(Greater cornu)
Thyroid cartilage
(Superior cornu)
False fold
Ventricle
True vocal fold
Pyriform sinus

Cricoid cartilage

Laryngeal
vestibule
Aryepiglottic
fold
Glottis
Cuneiform
cartilage

Corniculate
cartilage

FIGURE 2.2k Entrance to Larynx,
Posterior View Behind Tongue
Illustration, looking at the larynx as though
standing behind a person and seeing through
the back of his or her neck.

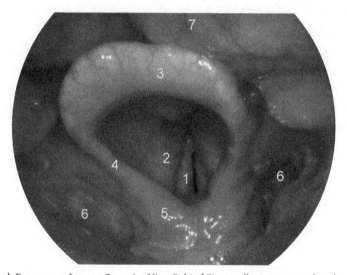

FIGURE 2.2l Entrance to Larynx, Posterior View Behind Tongue (laryngoscopy photo)
This photo shows a nasendoscope's view of the larynx but is flipped to simulate peering into the laryngeal vestibule.
1. True vocal fold (left). 2. False vocal fold (left). 3. Epiglottis. 4. Aryepiglottic fold (left side of the aryepiglottic sphincter). 5. Arytenoid cartilage (left). 6. **Pyriform sinuses** (right and left). 7. Base of tongue.

extends from either side of the bump and curves toward the back of the neck, creating a shield to protect the vocal folds behind it. The shield is approximately 3.5 cm across and 1.5 cm from the notch down, closed at the front and open toward the back of the neck.[2]

---

[2] Measurements taken by the author during cadaver **dissection** observations at The Ohio State University and from cadaver prosections used for the author's class at Michigan State University Gross Anatomy Lab.

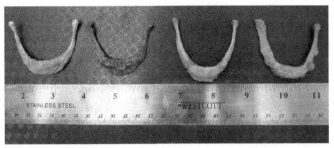

FIGURE 2.2m Hyoid Bone Samples
Samples of hyoid bones from cadavers show some of the variety in hyoid bone shapes.

Note: Hyoid literally means upsilon shaped, a capital Y and small υ in Greek. Upsilon literally means simple u and is the letter from which U and V came. Hyoid bones are often asymmetrical and vary greatly in shape, from a horseshoe with sides that curve slightly in, to a U-shape with straight sides, to more of a spread V-shape. (See Figure 2.2m.)

N. Papadopoulos, G. Lykaki-Anastopoulou, and E. Alvanidou. "The Shape and Size of the Human Hyoid Bone and a Proposal for an Alternative Classification." *Journal of Anatomy* 163 (1989): 163.

At the bottom of the thyroid cartilage, you'll discover another bump. You're feeling the front of the cricoid cartilage. The cricoid is like a signet or class ring with a 6-mm-wide band at the front that widens gradually to 2.5 cm where the signet or stone would be toward the back of the neck. It serves as the base of the larynx and is the only part of the larynx's framework that is not open at the back. (See Figure 2.2d.)

Note: The hyoid is the top-most portion of the larynx and the cricoid is the bottom-most portion of the larynx.

Note: We use "the back of the neck" as an easy point of reference for you to visualize how this anatomy sits inside your body. However, most of the neck is made up of bone or spine and your larynx takes up only a little space at the very front of the neck. (See Figure 2.2g.)

We can't touch or feel what lies behind these bumps, nor can we easily obtain a view on our own. The vocal folds extend horizontally in a "V" inside the larynx. If you had a very bright light and a small mirror that wouldn't steam up, you could stick your tongue out and peer behind and below your tongue to see this "V." (See Figures 2.2j, 2.2k, and 2.2l.) The space or opening of the "V" is called the **glottis**. The point of the "V" where the folds come together is called the **anterior commissure**. The anterior commissure attaches to the inside of the thyroid cartilage, just behind and below the thyroid notch at the front of the neck. The two arms of the "V" attach to the inside points of two pyramid-shaped

arytenoid cartilages perched atop the signet portion of the cricoid toward the back of the neck. The pyramids are about the size of blueberries and are like small stretched-out Hershey's Kisses or elf hats in shape.

We've been talking about looking down on the vocal folds and seeing them as two bands forming a "V" from above. However, if you were able to slice off the back portion of the larynx and look at the vocal folds from the back of the neck, you would see their depth. (See Figure 2.2e.)

The inner edge of each fold curves around, sloping downward and tapering underneath, blending in and becoming continuous with the cricothyroid membrane on the inside of the thyroid cartilage wall. (See Figure 2.2f.) The overall shape of each fold has the appearance of an exaggerated airplane wing. If you draw a question mark on a piece of paper and its mirror image to the right, you'll have an approximate outline of their shape. The biggest differences are that the shape of the free vibrating lips or edges (the upper curve of the question mark) is sharper on the vocal fold and the lower portion of the fold is not a sudden drop-off but tapers down gradually.

Still looking through the back of the neck, another pair of folds would be especially apparent just above the vocal folds. These are commonly known as the false vocal folds. They run parallel alongside and just above each true vocal fold. The space between the true and false folds is called the **ventricle**. A membranous sac called the **laryngeal saccule** extends up from the ventricle, separating the false fold from the inside of the thyroid cartilage wall. (See Figure 2.2e.)

You may be picturing the vocal folds taking up the entire inside of the neck. Actually, your vocal folds are incredibly tiny and they, as well as their surrounding cartilages, hardly extend beyond the front-most portion of the neck. Adult male vocal folds can span 17 to 25 mm in length (average 6 to 9 mm thick) and adult female vocal folds 12.5 to 17.5 mm (average 5 to 7 mm thick). To visualize this, draw a "V" across a quarter for a low bass voice, a "V" across a nickel for the average male, and a "V" across a dime for a female with a high soprano voice. (See Figure 2.2h.)

The cricoid encircles the top of the windpipe or **trachea**, so the vocal folds' "V" sits just over the pipe's opening. If you gently explore the dip at the front base of your neck just below the cricoid, you may make out a couple of the trachea's rings of cartilage. Eighteen to twenty-two C-shaped rings of cartilage hold open the otherwise membranous and muscular tracheal tube. The cartilages are closed at the front and open toward the back of the neck to allow flexibility and expansion of the tube during heavy breathing. (See Figure 2.2d.) The roughly 13.5-cm (5.4-inch) tube can elongate as much as 2 cm on deep inhalation.[3] You might be surprised to learn that the

[3] Paul Stark, "Radiology of the Trachea," ed. Nestor L. Muller. UpToDate, last modified October 13, 2009, http://www.uptodate.com/patients/content/topic.do?topicKey=~5CfPy6YkRYbqVI, accessed December 11, 2010.

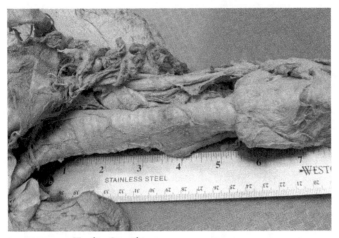

FIGURE 2.2n Trachea Length
Cadaver prosection shows the trachea to be about 13.5 cm/5.4 inches in length.

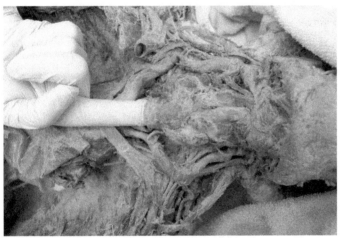

FIGURE 2.2o Trachea Diameter
Cadaver dissection shows one trachea's diameter in relation to an index finger.

trachea's inner diameter is only about 2 cm.[4,5] All air passing in and out of your body does so through a pipe that would accommodate little more than your index finger! (See Figures 2.2n and 2.2o.)

---

[4] The internal diameter measures roughly 1.9 cm from front to back and 2.0 cm from side to side in adult males and 1.6 cm × 1.7 cm for adult females. See Eamann Breatnach, Gypsy C. Abbott, and Robert G. Fraser, "Dimensions of the Normal Human Trachea," *American Journal of Roentgenology* 141 (May 1983): 903.

[5] The average tracheal width was 20.9 mm for men and 16.9 mm for women. See Jay B. Brodsky, Alex Macario, and James B.D. Mark, "Tracheal Diameter Predicts Double-Lumen Tube Size: A Method for Selecting Left Double-Lumen Tubes," *Anesthesia & Analgesia* 82, no. 4 (April 1996): 861.

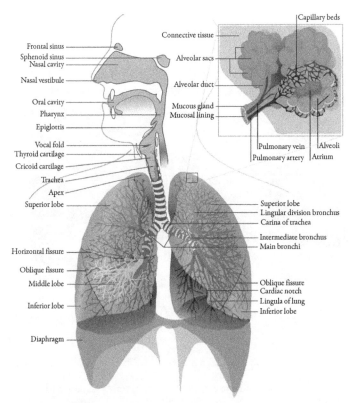

Frontal sinus
Sphenoid sinus
Nasal cavity
Nasal vestibule
Oral cavity
Pharynx
Epiglottis
Vocal fold
Thyroid cartilage
Cricoid cartilage
Trachea
Apex
Superior lobe
Horizontal fissure
Oblique fissure
Middle lobe
Inferior lobe
Diaphragm

Connective tissue
Alveolar sacs
Alveolar duct
Mucous gland
Mucosal lining
Capillary beds
Pulmonary vein
Pulmonary artery
Alveoli
Atrium

Superior lobe
Lingular division bronchus
Carina of trachea
Intermediate bronchus
Main bronchi
Oblique fissure
Cardiac notch
Lingula of lung
Inferior lobe

FIGURE 2.2p Respiratory System
The esophagus is shown but not labeled here. It is the tube just behind the trachea and is visible because the figure's head and neck are turned. (This diagram offers more lung detail than what is discussed in this text.)

> Note: The trachea is not a perfect cylinder. The trachea is flat on its **posterior** side across the opening of the C-shaped cartilages. Therefore, the diameter from front to back is slightly smaller than that from side to side.

At the bottom of the trachea, the tube divides into two tubes called bronchi. One enters the right lung and the other enters the left. Each bronchus splits off into hair-thin tubes inside the lung called bronchioles, which each ends in air sacs called alveoli. The overall appearance is similar to a sprig of curly parsley in each lung. A healthy adult lung is 850 g in men and 750 g in women[6] (about one and a half to two pounds), is spongy, and is slightly smaller than a football. When completely drained and dried, lungs are light and resemble natural sea sponges.[7] (See Figures 2.2p and 2.2q.)

---

[6] Gerald Baum, et al., eds., *Textbook of Pulmonary Diseases*, Vol. 1 (Philadelphia: Lippincott-Raven, 1998), 23.

[7] Personal observations made by the author from cadaver prosections used in the author's class at Michigan State University Gross Anatomy Lab.

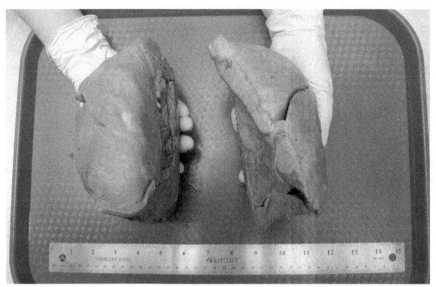

FIGURE 2.2q Lung Size
Prosected adult lungs taken from a cadaver can be compared to an American football in size.

Note: A lung taken from the cadaver of a heavy smoker is noticeably darker and less spongy as well, stiffened by tar that has coated the tiny channels for air with long-term smoke inhalation.

Although you can't directly touch the lungs, you can feel the protective ribcage that surrounds and protects them. Find your flat breastbone or sternum where the ribs connect in the front. Follow the ribs around your sides and to the back where they connect to the spine. If you were able to hold your ribs, you would be holding literally a cage of bone. At the top of this cage are your collarbones (clavicles). The top of each lung reaches the clavicles. Now picture holding this cage in front of you and looking down into the cage from above. The floor of the cage is a sheet of muscle that domes upward into the cage like an upside-down salad bowl. This unpaired muscle is the second-largest muscle in the body and is called the **diaphragm**. The "rim" of the bowl connects in the front to a piece of cartilage at the very bottom of the sternum (called the xiphoid **process**) to the spine in the back and along the bottom ribs all the way around the ribcage. The dome portion of the bowl touches the bottoms of the lungs inside the cage. The diaphragm neatly separates the light and airy lung cavity from the heavier gut cavity filled with stomach and intestines below. All that sits above is considered the chest cavity or **thoracic cavity**, and all that lies below is referred to as the abdominal cavity.

Note: The largest muscle in the body is the gluteus maximus—the muscle making up the main portion of your bum.

Note: Muscles that connect to bones and cartilages are called **skeletal muscles**. Different from **smooth muscles** that work alone, such as the heart and esophagus, skeletal muscles work in pairs. One relaxes so that its partner may contract. This paired relationship is called **muscular antagonism**. The diaphragm and the **transverse arytenoid muscle** are unique in that they are the only *unpaired* skeletal muscles in the body.

The floor of the abdominal cavity is the pelvic bone, which cradles the pile of water balloon–like organs (a.k.a. **viscera** or guts) below the diaphragm and between the hips.[8] This bone is a bit like a right-side-up bowl that tilts slightly forward so that the water balloons are freer to fill and shift against the soft front wall of your belly.

2.3 THE BASIC MECHANICS

The vocal folds are about 1 cm deep[9] and, like a layered dessert, composed of many differently textured layers. To virtually navigate these layers, you may find it helpful to take the mirrored question marks you drew earlier and draw several increasingly smaller question marks to the side of each. We are going to move into the folds from the outermost layer in. (See Figure 2.2e, detail.) The outermost layer of the folds is a very thin (only three to five microscopic cells thick) transparent layer like raw egg white called the **epithelium**. This layer gives hydrated folds their wet sheen. The next layer in from the epithelium is the thinnest layer of the vocal folds called the **basement membrane**. It's attached to the epithelium and separates the epithelium from another transparent layer below called the superficial layer of the **lamina propria**. A combination of tiny blood vessels (**capillaries**); elastic, springy tissues; and a gelatinous fluid, the superficial layer of the lamina propria allows the vocal folds to **vibrate** beautifully. Together, the epithelium, basement membrane, and superficial lamina propria make up the "cover" of the folds.

Moving inward and deeper, the next two layers are called the **intermediate** lamina propria and deep lamina propria. They are composed of tissues like microscopic soft rubber

---

[8] The comparison of abdominal viscera to water balloons comes from Scott McCoy, *Your Voice: An Inside View* (Princeton, NJ: Inside View Press, 2004), 115.

[9] Depth as measured from the vocal fold's upper lateral attachment along the inside thyroid cartilage wall to the bottom of its tapered underside along the inside thyroid cartilage wall. The "bottom" is where the vocal fold epithelium switches to respiratory tract epithelium. The division can be seen by an actual line called the inferior arcuate.

bands and strands of cotton, respectively.[10] These layers are not completely distinct from each other. They interweave where they meet in the middle. Together, they are referred to as the "transitional layer" of the vocal fold and make up the **vocal ligament** that gives the folds some structural support. This ligament is a short cord of tough tissue like any other ligament in the body such as in the knee or elbow, but much tinier. It firmly connects the vocal fold from the inside of the thyroid cartilage to the arytenoid cartilage. (See Figure 2.2i.)

Further in past the ligament lies the densest and deepest layer of the vocal folds, a muscular layer generally referred to as the **thyroarytenoid muscles** (see Figure 2.2i). The thyroarytenoids extend from the thyroid to the arytenoid inside each vocal fold. The muscle is made up of two distinct bands that run inside each vocal fold:

The **medial** thyroarytenoid muscle (a.k.a. the vocalis) runs nearest to the vibrating edge and makes up the body or bulk of the vibrating portion of the vocal fold.

The **lateral** thyroarytenoid muscle (a.k.a. the thyromuscularis) runs just to the outside and slightly **inferior** to the vocalis.

As the folds vibrate for **phonation**, the looser outside cover rhythmically slips and slides over the stiffer and denser inner layers, making the folds look like symmetrical waves in water. We call the motion of the cover over the ligament and muscular layer of the fold a "**cover wave**."[11]

Note: Many voice and medical professionals use "**mucosal wave**" to refer to the vocal fold's vibratory motion generated in sound production. Calling this wave "mucosal" is somewhat inaccurate, however, because the wave does not involve the entire **mucosa**. All mucosa throughout the body is made up of an epithelium, a basement membrane, and a lamina propria. The folds adduct and phonation begins, setting the folds into motion and generating a wave in the loose layers of each vocal fold. The epithelium, basement membrane, and superficial layer of the lamina propria are the "waving" layers. The two deeper layers of the lamina propria are thicker connective tissues that are not part of this wave-like motion, but rather adhere to the vocalis muscle underneath and form the firmer "body" of the vocal fold. Because the superficial layer with the attached epithelium is the "cover" layer, the "wave" is more appropriately called the cover wave.

The two fleshy pink false folds each contain some muscle and a ligament called the **vestibular ligament** and are covered in mucosa. We have observed that there are two ways the false folds come closer together (**medialize**); one is passive and one is not. When

---

[10] Minoru Hirano, "Vocal Mechanisms in Singing: Laryngological and Phoniatric Aspects," *The Journal of Voice* 2, no.1 (1988): 52.

[11] "Cover wave" is a term coined by the authors, who hope to replace the traditional but technically incorrect term "mucosal wave" when referring to the vibratory motion of the cover over the body of the true vocal fold.

the false fold muscles contract, the false folds squeeze closer together. They contract and completely close when you hold your breath, swallow, clear your throat, cough, or make **glottal onsets** (e.g., "uh oh"). However, the false folds can remain passive and be squeezed together by surrounding muscular tissues, as we will talk more about later when we discuss "twang." (See 9.2 How Voice Specialists See Your Instrument.)

Note: The idea of the vocal folds having a "body" and a "cover" was first introduced by a scientist named Minoru **Hirano** to explain simply how the folds' layers behave during vibration. He published his body-cover theory in 1974. Hirano's theory does not address a transitional layer and divides body and cover differently than we do. Hirano's "body" includes only the very stiffest, densest layers: the *deep* layer of the lamina propria and the muscles in the vocal folds. His "cover" refers to the epithelium (and basement membrane), the superficial layer, and the *intermediate* layer of the lamina propria. The use of "cover" and "body" is inconsistent in the literature. Some use "cover" to refer only to the epithelium and basement membrane. Others use it like Hirano. Still others use it like we do to refer to the superficial, more flexible layers that present the most movement during vibration. Each model attempts to shed light on the complex roles the layers play during vibration.

As described earlier, the vocal folds span the airway, connecting in the front of the neck behind the Adam's apple and at the back to the arytenoid cartilages. The arytenoid cartilages sit atop the cricoid ring like a saddle on a horse, creating a unique pair of joints that can slide and pivot, as well as rock forward and backward. These cricoarytenoid joint motions swivel to open, close, and tense the vocal folds to varying degrees. The vocal folds are in their relaxed, completely open (**abducted**) position when you breathe and completely closed (**adducted**) under the false folds when you hold your breath. The true vocal folds forcefully adduct, drawing the false folds with them when you clear your throat or cough. They **approximate** or come close together to make an [h] sound. They also approximate to vibrate when you decide to make a sound. The air coming from your lungs interacts with your vibrating vocal folds to create the buzz-like sound wave that travels through your **resonating cavities** (**vocal tract**) and out of your mouth. (See the Bernoulli Effect in 2.4 The Many Functions of the Larynx.)

The true vocal folds are pulled longer when the thyroid cartilage tilts down from the cricoid. Remember that the folds are attached to the thyroid cartilage at the front of the neck and to the arytenoids sitting on the cricoid toward the back of the neck. The cricoid sits stationary on the top of the trachea, but the thyroid cartilage has some mobility due to its inferior horns (two lower protrusions), which form a joint on either side of the cricoid (cricothyroid joints). (See Figure 2.2d.) A muscle on both sides of the larynx (called the **cricothyroid muscle**) extends from the outside wall of the cricoid cartilage and attaches to the inner side wall of the thyroid cartilage. (See Figure 2.2c.) When the muscle contracts, it pulls the thyroid cartilage, tipping it down in the front. Because the vocal folds are fixed at the arytenoids on the cricoid, they are elongated by this contraction.

Note: You may be confused to hear the singular "cricothyroid muscle" used when referring to a muscle that exists on both sides of the larynx. Although arms, legs, lungs, arytenoid cartilages, vocal folds, and many other body parts are referred to in the plural, medical literature assumes *symmetry* when referring to nerves and muscles and often uses singular names! This can be confusing until you get to know anatomy better. The descriptions offered in this manual aim to dispel confusion as each anatomical part is introduced.

The air that powers the vocal fold vibrations comes up from the lungs. It may surprise you to learn that the lungs are not muscles. In fact, they are soft tissue and have no muscular properties whatsoever! They rely completely on the diaphragm and rib muscles to inflate them and on the rib and abdominal muscles to deflate them. These special actions occur because the lungs are encased by a thin layer of fluid called the pleural sac. The wetness of this sac creates an airtight seal that adheres the lungs to the surrounding ribcage walls and diaphragm floor. The adhesive effect is so strong that when the diaphragm lowers and the ribs expand out and up, they draw the lungs down and out, pulling air into the lungs.

When our diaphragm contracts, it lowers and flattens slightly, pressing down onto the organs in our abdomen. The water balloon–like organs that make up our gut cannot be squished smaller, only displaced.[12] Because they are cradled in a bowl-like pelvis underneath and trapped by the spine and big muscles in back, the organs will get "smooshed" down and out, as long as we are not holding our bellies in. A belly that bulges out or a waistband that feels tighter on inhalation indicates a breath that has involved a lot of diaphragmatic contraction and abdominal relaxation.

On exhalation, the diaphragm relaxes from its contracted position back up to its upside-down bowl shape. The exhalation muscles—the abdominal wall muscles and some of the muscles between the ribs—contract to fully expel or use up the air in the lungs.

All laryngeal sensation and movement input is delivered from the brain to the larynx via the **superior laryngeal nerve** (**SLN**) and the **recurrent laryngeal nerve** (**RLN**). These nerves are not connected to the brain directly, however. They branch off of a major nerve (their "parent" nerve) stemming from the brain called the **vagus**. The vagus starts at the brain's medulla oblongata at the top of the neck, inside the base of the skull. Like all other **cranial** nerves, the vagus is paired, meaning that one vagus emerges from the right

---

[12] McCoy, *Your Voice*, 115.

side of the brain and another emerges from the left side of the brain. Each vagus goes out a hole on either side of the skull called the jugular foramen and begins its journey downward to innervate its respective side of the body.

Note: It has long been debated by singers—including top **voice pedagogues**—whether the diaphragm is a voluntary or involuntary muscle. Technically, the muscle itself is neither. The *nervous system's control* over a muscle is voluntary or involuntary. Unlike the cardiac muscle of the heart and smooth muscles of the trachea, uterus, and intestines, which all contract spontaneously and involuntarily, the diaphragm is skeletal muscle (suspended by the bottom ribs), suggesting that like all skeletal muscle the diaphragm's **innervation** is voluntary. However, the diaphragm is unique in two ways. The first is that, although a skeletal muscle, its innervation is primarily *involuntary*. The diaphragm is controlled by the brainstem (a.k.a. under "normal control"), which handles all of the body's primitive functions needed to stay alive (such as blood circulation and digestion). The brainstem innervates the diaphragm via the phrenic nerve, causing it to contract for passive breathing, sneezes, and hiccups, or when it senses our body's need for oxygen (yawning, gasping after holding our breath or running, and similarly contracting to draw air in after speaking or singing a long phrase or sustained pitch). The second way the diaphragm is unique is that we have direct voluntary control over its contraction as well! The cortical control of our brain's thinking cortex can *override* the normal control of the brainstem and send a direct voluntary impulse to the phrenic nerve when we want to alter the way we breathe. Our cortex will perform an override when we *choose* to inhale, take deeper or shallower breaths, or determine how to release those breaths on exhalation. Some of the many ways we choose to breathe and voluntarily employ the diaphragm are panting or singing staccato, holding the breath or sustaining a long pitch, tanking up to blow out lots of candles or preparing for a sforzando, and deciding to take a small catch-breath or "lift" within a phrase.

Scott McCoy. *Your Voice: An Inside View* (Princeton, NJ: Inside View Press, 2004), 89. Richard Miller. *Training Soprano Voices* (New York: Oxford University Press, 2000), 38.Shirley Emmon's discussion of diaphragmatic control on the website: http://www.shirlee-emmons.com/breath_management.html. Accessed June 23, 2012.

Note: Vagus is Latin for "wandering"—think of the word "vagabond," which shares the same root. Because this nerve has a long route from your brain all the way down to your colon, it is well named!

The vagus nerve is one large bundle composed of smaller prepackaged bundles of neuronal fibers (like the SLN and RLN) that are each wrapped like telephone wire in layers of connective tissue. In other words, there are prepackaged bundles of fibers that are then packaged together with more connective tissue to form the vagus nerve.

Shortly after leaving the skull and near to the **carotid artery**, the vagus (on each side) gives off—like a section of string cheese pulled almost off the cheese stick—the SLN. The SLN is a short branch, as thin as a strand of hair. The external SLN (right and left) travels along the sides of the neck, innervating the cricothyroid muscle on the *outside* of the larynx so that the vocal folds can change pitch. The SLN then sends a branch into the larynx by going through the hyothyroid membrane. (See Figure 2.2c.) This internal SLN provides sensation in the laryngeal linings down to the vocal fold level (**supraglottis**). It creates the tickle you feel when it detects an irritant, for instance, and provokes you to cough.

After the vagus nerve gives off the SLN branch, the vagus continues down the neck, just behind the carotid artery and into the chest, where it gives off the recurrent laryngeal nerve before following the esophagus down through the diaphragm to the stomach. The right RLN remains bundled with the vagus, traveling down to just behind the collarbone (a.k.a. clavicle) in the upper chest, where it branches off and circles around the **subclavian artery**. The longer left RLN stays bundled with the vagus until it descends farther into the chest near to the heart, where it branches

---

Note: The RLN earned the name "recurrent" because it takes such an indirect, roundabout route to the larynx. The oddly indirect paths of the RLN make it susceptible to damage during neck (e.g., thyroid, carotid artery) and chest (e.g., heart, lung) surgeries, which can result in nerve-related problems in the larynx.

Note: Many scientists think that the RLN originally traveled directly from the brain, past the heart, to the gills of our earliest fish-like ancestors because that is the route it takes in fish today. Over time, as ancestors of mammals developed and slowly evolved away from their fish ancestors, the larynx and lungs eventually replaced gills, and necks lengthened. The orderly routes of the earliest ancestors' nerves still observed in modern fish and sharks became messy. If mammals were created from scratch rather than evolving from fish-like ancestors, you would think that the vagus nerve would give off the RLN as it approaches the larynx. Instead, the vagus just gets longer, while the RLN branch, on the wrong side of the heart to reach the newly formed larynx, must travel under the aorta before it makes an absurdly long journey up to enervate laryngeal muscles.

Richard Dawkins. "History Written All Over Us." *The Greatest Show on Earth* (New York: Free Press, 2009), 360–364.

off and loops under the **aorta** before proceeding back up to the larynx. The recurrent laryngeal nerve branches (right and left) supply all of the larynx's muscles, other than the cricothyroid mentioned previously.

2.4 THE MANY FUNCTIONS OF THE LARYNX

The larynx is your instrument, but its significance goes beyond just producing sound. The larynx plays three very important roles in your body. The larynx assists in swallowing (**deglutition**) and prevents anything but air from entering the windpipe and lungs. The larynx closes and elevates during swallowing to assist in the passage of food. Swallowing and airway protection are so important that the larynx is prepared to launch into action at the first sign of a potentially hazardous situation. A special type of **mucous membrane** or mucosa called **nonkeratinizing stratified squamous cell epithelium**—whew!—lines most of the larynx. (See note below.) This membrane is composed of ultra-sensitive cells that trigger a cough or a throat clear when any substance outside of their normal environment touches them (such as food, dust, an inhaled insect, or very cold air). These sensory cells increase in number the closer they reside to the vocal folds, making the lining increasingly sensitive. If a "foreign substance" touches near the vocal folds, the cells will signal for your larynx to spasm or close (**laryngospasm**). The laryngeal muscles will fiercely contract, the **epiglottis** will snap shut over the windpipe (trachea), and the vocal folds will pull together to form a protective shield over the trachea. This spasm usually resolves within a few seconds, but if the foreign substance hits the vocal folds, the spasm can be so severe that both speaking and breathing can be stopped for up to two minutes before the vocal folds slowly reopen. In very rare cases, the spasm is not released and has been known to cause death. Fortunately, the lining is equipped to sense a foreign substance well before it nears the vocal folds, making a spasm a rare event.

Note: The lining of the larynx is all mucosa. Mucosa forms a protective barrier between our bodies and the environment. However, not all mucosa is the same. If you were able to see the entire larynx under a microscope, you'd notice differences in the cellular make-up, or the **histology,** of the mucosa at a couple points on the larynx. At this microscopic cellular level you'd see that the mucosa that lines the false folds and ventricle has a respiratory epithelium called pseudostratified ciliated columnar epithelium. This is the same epithelium found in the nose, trachea, and bronchi that secretes **mucus** to trap foreign particles and uses tiny hair-like cilia cells to wave the particles away from the airway. Respiratory epithelium at the laryngeal level makes sense; the larynx is the entrance to the trachea, after all, and therefore part of the respiratory system. The rest of the larynx is lined in mucosa that has a nonkeratinizing stratified squamous cell epithelium.

The larynx's second role is that it allows you to hold your breath. Your false and true vocal folds close over the trachea to prevent air from escaping. The trapped air provides a pressurized resistance for you to lean on during heavy lifting and pushing, as in defecation and childbirth. This resistance is properly referred to as a **Valsalva maneuver** or **thoracic fixation**, meaning that the thoracic cavity, commonly known as the chest, is stabilized.

Note: Some texts also refer to thoracic fixation as abdominal fixation.

Lastly, and only when not engaged in one of its other roles, the larynx can be used to produce sound. To produce sound, laryngeal muscles contract to adduct the vocal folds. As the vocal folds come together, air travels up from the lungs through the trachea to meet the narrowed folds. As the air passes between the narrowed folds, they get pulled together and vibration begins. It is this vibration that results in sound. You may wonder, "Why are the folds being pulled together by air passing between them?" We attribute this phenomenon to the **Bernoulli Effect**, which explains that moving air has less density than stagnant air. You may have experienced something similar to the Bernoulli Effect in your shower. The air inside the shower is moving faster than the air outside the shower due to the movement created from the running water. As a result, the shower curtain pulls away from the sides of the tub and into the shower, resulting in an annoying bathing experience.[13]

Likewise, when air passes between the narrowed and flexible vocal folds, the drop in air pressure pulls the folds together.[14] To illustrate this concept further, try holding one edge of a piece of paper just under your bottom lip and blowing air out of your mouth above the paper. The paper will travel toward the moving air. Now try blowing between two pieces of paper. The pages will come together and blow apart, again and again, creating a buzz. Vocal folds behave similarly as air passes between them. After the folds are pulled together, air pressure builds up below the closed vocal folds (a.k.a. **subglottal** pressure) and then blows them apart. The folds then spring back together (**elastic recoil**) and remain together until the subglottal pressure builds again and the cycle repeats itself. This opening and closing over air produce vibrations that make sound. Each vibration (one opening and one closing) of the vocal folds is called one *cycle* of phonation or a vibratory cycle. Each vibratory cycle is also called a **period.**

---

[13] This is a simplified example of phonation and does not really account for the complexity of this process as the vocal folds are always under some neural control and are not merely passive participants with varying airflow.

[14] Often the vocal folds are described as being "sucked" together as a result of the Bernoulli Effect. However, scientists and mathematicians prefer the term "pulled" or "brought." The word "sucked" implies air pressure that is literally pulling in (as in sucking in through a straw). Because nothing is actually sucking air from between the folds, this term does not accurately describe how they're coming together.

A breathy tone or a nonbreathy tone is determined by how long and how completely the vocal folds close during each cycle of vibration. Each moment that the vocal folds close during phonation, air pressure temporarily builds up below the vocal folds. This pressure is referred to as subglottal pressure. The longer the vocal folds remain in the closed portion (a.k.a. closed phase) of each vibratory cycle, the more the air pressure builds underneath the folds (more subglottal pressure), and a less breathy tone is the result. Conversely, a breathy tone is the result of less air building up below the folds (less subglottal pressure) due to the folds staying in a more "open" position that allows a greater amount of air to escape with each cycle.

> Note: When we discuss phase closure, we are comparing open phase to closed phase or the ratio of time the glottis is open to the time the glottis is closed within each vibratory cycle.

Subglottal pressure also determines the loudness or quietness of the sound. Each time the vocal folds close during a cycle of phonation, air pressure builds in the trachea below. You can think of the vocal folds sitting on top of the trachea like a valve. A valve or nozzle on the end of a garden hose can be tightened to constrict a great flow of water so that the water can reach farther. Similarly, the folds' deepest layer is made up of muscles (thyroarytenoid muscles) that bulk during contraction, tensing the folds to create more and more subglottal pressure. The tighter the valve is, the greater the subglottal pressure and the louder the tone. (See 14.11 To What Extent Is a Great Voice Determined by Vocal Physiology?)

> Note: It is very difficult to maintain the same volume as we're running out of breath. Some people will talk or sing until they run out of breath and have to induce muscular tension in the larynx to maintain enough subglottal pressure to finish. Over time, such vocal tension can become habitual and problematic. (See 10.15 Muscle Tension Dysphonia.) Classical singers work hard to master the motor skill needed to slowly and evenly contract and then relax the thyroarytenoid muscles with a vocalise called "*messa di voce.*" In this exercise, the singer practices seamlessly transitioning and very gradually, from a soft sound to a louder sound and then back to a soft sound, all on one pitch and one breath. The exercise is one of the most difficult vocalises and requires a coordinated increase and decrease in vocal fold thickness (or mass) with a well-supported, steady increase and decrease of breath.

The pitch produced depends on the length of the vocal folds and the number of times the vocal folds vibrate per second, but it's not simple! Consider what you may already know about how pitch relates to size: A long thick piano string produces a low sound, and a short thin one makes a high sound; a cello has a lower, deeper sound than a violin; and a flute is lower in sound than a piccolo. Similarly, a male's vocal folds, because they tend to be longer and fatter than those of a female's, tend to produce a fundamentally lower and deeper sound quality. However, the vocal folds have the ability to vary their length and thickness. The way they go about changing pitches relates best with a rubber band or guitar string. If you stretch a rubber band long and taut or tighten the fret of a guitar string and pluck, the band and string will produce a higher sound than if you give either some slack and pluck. Both the band and string have undergone changes in thickness. A thinner, tauter string has less mass per unit, and vibrations will pass more quickly through it than a looser, fatter string. Similarly, your folds are pulled longer, thinner, and tauter the higher you sing. The wave of vibration passing through the tauter cover moves to the **medial edge** of the folds. The cover's flexibility diminishes as the folds continue to lengthen, and the vibrations pass through more and more quickly, creating higher and higher frequencies. For very high notes, only the medial and front-most portion of the cover vibrates. As you descend in pitch, the folds grow shorter and fatter, until the entire cover freely waves in vibration. The skin on the top of your hand may be compared to the vocal fold cover to help you picture how the cover works. When your hand is relaxed, the skin on top is very pliable. When the hand is flexed to make a fist, however, the skin becomes very taut and flexibility is diminished.

3

The Singer as an Athlete

SINGING IS NOT aerobic exercise. In other words, singing does not increase your heart rate and burn fat, nor does it help you lose weight. Singing is *an*aerobic exercise. Because anaerobic means "without oxygen," using the term to describe singing seems counterintuitive. We need air to sing! But anaerobic exercise does not mean an exercise done without breathing. Instead, anaerobic describes exercises, like singing and lifting weights, that do not sustain activity long enough for the body's tissues to begin heavily demanding oxygen. Aerobic exercises, on the other hand, such as running and swimming, cause you to involuntarily breathe heavily because the body's tissues are demanding oxygen.

Anaerobic exercise also places intense demands on muscles and forces them to develop to meet those demands. Singing places intense demands on muscles in the head, neck, and torso. Singers use vocalises, or voice exercises, designed to isolate, coordinate, and strengthen specific muscle contractions until they've developed the fine muscle control needed to evenly crescendo and decrescendo, shift smoothly between chest and head registers, mix registers for belting, or even quickly alternate between the registers for yodeling! Additionally, the demands made by healthy, well-trained singing help to develop excellent posture, efficient breath control, and, some say, expanded vital capacity in the lungs.

Breath support, or controlling the rate of exhalation, is a good example of anaerobic exercise. We can control the rate at which we exhale by contracting muscles in the abdomen and chest. Perhaps the most complex example of breath support is the type used by classical singers. Breaths that rely heavily on both abdominal and chest musculature are considered optimal for classical singing. These breaths are aptly called thoracic-abdominal or combination breaths. When classical singers inhale, they expand the rib cage and relax the abdominal muscles, allowing the diaphragm to press the viscera below it down. Basically they get a big chest and a fat tummy! While they're singing, classical singers work to maintain the pressures created during inhalation: the outward expansion of the ribs and the pressure of the diaphragm on the viscera below. By striving to maintain these pressures, classical singers are able to stave off the inevitable contraction of the abdominal muscles and prolong exhalation. (See **appoggio** in 15.3 Vocabulary.) Additionally, the abdominal relaxation involved in combination breathing actually helps to lower the larynx, resulting in a richer, deeper timbre stylistically suited for opera and Shakespearean speaking.

Other types of singing, for example, pop, rock, country, and some musical theater, require breaths that involve mostly chest expansion and less abdominal distension than classical singing. This helps create a slightly higher laryngeal position to achieve the stylistically desired sound. The breathing used for these styles is called chest breathing, thoracic breathing, or **costal** breathing. Singers in these styles maintain ribcage expansion and use chest muscles to control the rate of exhalation and resist the ribcage's collapse. Although costal breathing does not offer as much control over the rate of exhalation as combination breathing, this is not usually a problem for belters who tend to sing in shorter phrases. Regardless of style, well-trained singers and speakers spend much time practicing controlled releases of exhalation to strengthen the muscles used for respiration. Over time, this practice potentially expands their lungs' vital capacity.

Note: We prefer to use the expression "combination breathing" when referring to the breath used by classical vocalists. Others refer to combination breathing as "balanced breathing" because it relies more equally than other types of breathing on both the abdominal and thoracic musculature. However, because some misunderstand the term "balanced" to imply that thoracic breathing isn't balanced, we choose not to use the term. Other common ways to describe combination breathing are "breathing with your diaphragm," "belly breathing," and "abdominal breathing," but because all breathing contracts the diaphragm *and* because breath doesn't enter the belly, these names just tend to be confusing!

Although lung size and respiratory muscle strength vary from person to person, the average adult is capable of inhaling and exhaling about four to five liters of air from his or her lungs. This is known as vital capacity.[1] During everyday, passive breathing, we circulate only about half a liter from our vital capacity for each breath. This is our **tidal volume**. Singing and dramatic speech interrupt natural, rhythmic breathing patterns and frequently require much more of our vital capacity to sing or dramatically speak a phrase. Different amounts of breath are inhaled to sing or speak, depending on the phrase to be spoken or sung.[2] A large breath is needed to create the necessary subglottal pressure for healthy projection, and a large breath is also needed to maintain consistent subglottal pressure over a very long phrase. As a result much of your vital capacity will regularly circulate while singing, belting, projecting speech, or delivering long soliloquies.

The combination breath used for classical singing is often mistakenly considered to be the breath that fills the lungs most completely. Actually, the high "clavicular" breaths that are brought on by aerobic exertion fill the lungs more.[3] This makes sense when you remember that aerobic exercise causes the body's tissues to demand oxygen and elicits involuntarily heavy breathing! Combination breaths may seem to draw the most air, because they allow us to speak and sing for the longest period of time without taking a breath. This benefit, however, has less to do with how much we've inhaled and more to do with the increased control (discussed earlier) that the combination breath gives over exhalation. Consider the awesome abdominal control needed to deliver the four to five liters over the lengthy single-breath phrases in "Der Hölle Rache kocht in meinem Herzen" from Mozart's *Die Zauberflöte*, Handel's "Eternal source," or Ochs's "Dank, sei dir, Herr." Such super control over muscles requires *strength*, not *air*, and is developed only through anaerobic exercise. While the combination breath offers greater control over exhalation, both costal and combination breathing offer the best support for their respective styles of phonation.

Note: Trained singers will often imagine they are *using* great amounts of breath to set the folds in motion for singing when in fact what they are really doing is *controlling* the exhalation of breath efficiently. Very little air is needed to get the folds vibrating.

---

[1] Leon Thurman et al., "Creating Breathflow for Skilled Speaking and Singing," in *Bodymind and Voice: Foundations of Voice Education*, ed. Leon Thurman and Graham Welch (Iowa City: National Center for Voice and Speech, 1997), 168.

[2] Many singers feel they need to try to fill the lungs completely to sing. They may "tank up" only to find that they have taken in too much air and have an abundance to exhale at the end of a phrase. Some never exhale the extra breath, and when they go to take the next breath, they "stack" the breath on top of the excess, inhaling more that isn't needed. "Loading" or overinflating the lungs for singing puts a lot of pressure against the underside of the vocal folds (subglottal pressure) and, depending on the phrase, may make it difficult to sing.
Think of preparing to jump over an obstacle, such as a fence. If the fence is high, you will choose to begin running from farther back than you would for a low fence in order to gain momentum. So should you not take the same amount of breath for every type of musical phrase.

[3] Scott McCoy, *Your Voice: An Inside View* (Princeton, NJ: Inside View Press, 2004), 94.

Note: You may hear the word "volume" used instead of "capacity" when referring to amounts the lungs can hold. Volume is what can be directly measured by scientists, whereas capacity is an amount estimated based on volume measurements. For instance, vital capacity is deduced from the amount of air the average person can exhale from his or her lungs. (See also **residual air**, **total lung capacity**, and **total lung volume** in 15.3 Vocabulary.)

What might be confusing when thinking about singing as being anaerobic is that "anaerobic" typically describes exercise that is done in short intense spurts (think jumps, sit-ups, push-ups, and weight lifting) to bulk muscle. Research has not been done, but we speculate that if we were to only use our voices to yell in short fortissimo outbursts, the thyroarytenoid muscles may begin to bulk. Laryngeal musculature, however, is not typically developed with short bursts of activity. Their long-term (lifelong!) work out of day-to-day phonation conditions them into long, thin muscles designed for endurance.

Although a well-trained singer's laryngeal anatomy will not get "ripped" à la Arnold Schwarzenegger, it often appears healthier overall with better vocal fold closure and more muscular balance, especially when compared with that of nonsingers. **Laryngologist** and coauthor of this manual Dr. Arick Forrest has found that because of the extreme range, fine motor control, and stamina their discipline demands, such distinctions are particularly evident in classically trained singers with the addition of highly elastic folds that elongate easily. Other genres of singing tend to predominantly employ the modal register (the same pitches used for speech) and don't necessarily use laryngeal musculature to its utmost capacity on a consistent basis.

For your voice to function optimally and gain endurance, you must follow a discipline of adequate sleep, nutrition, hydration, muscular conditioning, and appropriate exercise.

3.2 SLEEP

Current research consistently demonstrates that seven to eight hours of sleep each night is vital for adults. The detrimental effects from a lack of sleep accumulated over days can equal the detrimental effects resulting from one to three days' total lack of sleep.[4] Studies show that getting less than seven hours of sleep each night (especially when frequent) can contribute to a shorter attention span, poor memory, obesity, increased blood pressure, heart disease, and shorter life span.[5] Jet lag is a common inconvenience among

---

[4] Siobhan Banks and David F. Dinges, "Behavioral and Physiological Consequences of Sleep Restriction," *Journal of Clinical Sleep Medicine* 3, no. 5 (August 15, 2007): 519.

[5] Banks and Dinges, "Behavioral and Physiological Consequences of Sleep Restriction," 526.

professional singers, because a career in singing can demand a lot of national and international traveling. If you're preparing to perform in a time zone with a two-hour difference or more, you may benefit by gradually adapting to the time zone well before you arrive. Acclimatize your practice, diet, and sleep patterns to the new schedule while at home three days before departure. Once at your destination, get as much natural light exposure as possible. Your body will more readily adjust and be ready to perform. Dr. Charles F. Ehret created a system that is used by Argonne's Division of Biological and Medical Research to assist travelers and shift workers (e.g., hospital clinicians and power plant operators) who must periodically reprogram their internal clocks. See Dr. Ehret's book, *Overcoming Jet Lag* (Berkeley, 1983), for specific recommendations on how to efficiently handle the shift.

3.3 NUTRITION

Like endurance athletes, singers need a wide variety of foods that are low in fat and high in carbohydrates and fiber. For optimum performance, never skip breakfast. By eating after eight or so hours of sleep, you are essentially breaking a fast (hence the word "breakfast") and should eat within two hours of waking.[6] Research has shown that breakfast skippers compromise their ability to concentrate, train less effectively, and perform suboptimally. You may experience less fatigue eating six small meals a day rather than two or three large ones.[7] Three meals and three light snacks may work for most to prevent fatigue and low blood sugars, but some may prefer three meals and one or two snacks as needed.[8] The goal is to maintain a balance between energy intake and energy burning. You may benefit by following something similar to an endurance athlete's recommended dietary regimen on the day of a two- to three-hour performance. Four hours before your performance, drink seventeen to twenty ounces of water. Three to four hours before your performance, eat a meal that is high in low-glycemic (low-sugar) carbohydrates and lean protein and low in fat and fiber.

Note: Avoiding fiber on the day of a performance is important only if you tend to get pre-performance jitters, because the fiber tends to worsen the condition and your butterflies may leave you in the bathroom instead of backstage!

---

[6] Esther Park, MS, RD, e-mail message to author, March 14, 2012.
[7] University of California at Berkeley, ed., *The New Wellness Encyclopedia* (Boston: Houghton Mifflin, 1995), 77–78.
[8] Esther Park, MS, RD, e-mail message to author, March 14, 2012.

Additionally, a high-carbohydrate, moderate-protein, low-fat, and low-fiber snack with five to ten ounces of water is recommended thirty minutes to an hour before the performance to enhance stamina and endurance.[9] Although many singers believe they should sing on an empty stomach, this type of pre-performance snack should not get in the way of taking full breaths and producing clean, clear sounds. Just be sure to choose your pre-performance snack wisely and don't overindulge! Although these recommendations are given, dietary guidelines are personal and should take into account existing health conditions such as **reflux** or obesity, possible genetic factors like risk for diabetes or heart disease, and general responses to the foods that are chosen. There are foods that simply do not "sit well" with some people and should not be consumed by them. Again, only you know what foods make you feel healthy and energetic long after the meal has been completed.

3.4 FOODS TO AVOID AND WHY

Caffeine is a stimulant and should be consumed conservatively, if at all, by singers. Aside from its potential to cause irritability and nervousness, it can irritate the bladder and give you the need to urinate more often. Study results suggest that the body can develop a tolerance to caffeine with regular consumption and not experience these effects. Studies have also shown that those who consume two to three eight-ounce cups of coffee after abstaining from caffeine for a period of days will need to urinate more often but not urinate more in quantity.[10] After reviewing and weighing the results of the literature, experts at the Mayo Clinic concluded that consuming more than 500 to 600 mg of caffeine has a diuretic effect and causes our bodies to lose water.[11,12] Until more is known, we suggest that you not drink too much caffeine. What you're really looking for to have a successful performance is *stability*. If you are not accustomed to caffeine, it is probably wise not to start consuming caffeine. As a serious singer, you need plenty of water. You are probably rarely seen without your water bottle and are likely urinating often enough without caffeine as it is!

Caffeinated substances differ in how much caffeine they contain. Even among coffees, caffeine amounts vary. An eight-ounce cup of caffeinated coffee typically has 100 mg of

[9] © Academy of Nutrition and Dietetics (formerly American Dietetic Association), Sports Nutrition Care Manual, Client Education > Endurance Athletes > Meal Planning Tips and Food Lists, last modified 2010, http://nutritioncaremanual.org/content.cfm?ncm_content_id=110785, accessed January 16, 2012. Reprinted with permission.

[10] R. J. Maughan and J. Griffin, "Caffeine Ingestion and Fluid Balance: A Review," *Journal of Human Nutrition and Dietetics* 16, no. 6 (2003): 411, doi:10.1046/j.1365–277X.2003.00477.x.

[11] Five hundred to six hundred milligrams of caffeine is roughly equivalent to forty to fifty-six ounces of coffee, depending on the brand, the concentration, and the freshness of the brewed pot.

[12] Katherine Zeratsky, "Caffeine: Is It Dehydrating or Not?" last modified August 21, 2009, *Nutrition and Healthy Eating,* http://www.mayoclinic.com/health/caffeinated-drinks/AN01661.

caffeine but, depending on the brand, the grind, and the type of bean, can have anywhere from 58 to 281 mg of caffeine![13]

Aside from coffee, caffeine and occasionally other **methylxanthines** (natural stimulants found in food) are found in black teas, green teas, white teas, many sodas, chocolate, energy drinks, some medications, and even some bottled water. Because caffeine cannot be completely removed from something that is naturally caffeinated, all "decaf" drinks contain some amount of caffeine. While they may be less of an issue, there are no regulations on how much caffeine must be removed for coffee to be considered decaffeinated. Caffeine in decaf coffee can range from 5 to 32 mg.[14] Water evaporation contributes, too; the older the pot of coffee (or tea), the higher the caffeine concentration. Herbal coffees and teas (e.g., mint, chamomile, hibiscus, and red "rooibos") are caffeine-free, meaning they never had caffeine to begin with. The Food and Drug Administration requires that all labels clearly indicate any ingredient, so if caffeine is in your drink, it should be listed on the label.

Studies show that alcohol, including beer and wine, will pull water from your body within the first three hours after drinking. Your body will begin to retain water six hours after drinking. This water retention response is your body's attempt at compensating for the fluid loss, and this effort to reestablish fluid balance or homeostasis can last up until the twelfth hour after ingesting alcohol. In other words, you may retain water for up to six hours.[15] Alcohol will dehydrate the vocal fold epithelium during the diuretic phase. We speculate that the period of retaining water may affect the superficial lamina propria and possibly cause the vocal folds to feel heavy with no positive effect on singing. While there isn't research to back up this speculation, we advise that you refrain from drinking alcohol twenty-four hours prior to performing to be safe.

Salt intake should be limited to a maximum of 2,300 mg (about one teaspoon) per day. Excess salt will not cause the vocal folds to retain water like it will to the rest of the body, but frequent excessive salt intake can contribute to their dehydration. To maintain homeostasis, the body uses water to pee out what it cannot use. Over time, a loss of water due to a high-salt diet will contribute to vocal fold dehydration.

---

[13] "Is It Really Decaf?" *Consumer Reports* (November 2007): 7, http://www.consumerreports.org/cro/food/beverages/coffee-tea/is -it-really decaffeinated-coffee-11–07/overview/decaf-coffee-ov.html, accessed November 24, 2010.

[14] "Is It Really Decaf?" 7.

[15] The Institute of Medicine (IOM) report reviewed research suggesting that although alcohol has a diuretic effect on the body within the first three hours after drinking, the body compensates by going into an antidiuretic mode of retaining water thereafter. After twenty-four hours the body exhibited no significant fluid loss: "… it appears that the effect of ethanol ingestion on increasing excretion of water appears to be transient and would not result in appreciable fluid losses over a 24-hr period." Institute of Medicine and Food and Nutrition Board, *Dietary Reference Intakes for Water, Potassium, Sodium, Chloride, and Sulfate* (Washington, DC: National Academies Press, 2004).

Sugar offers a quick energy rush that will soon after leave you feeling tired. On the day of a performance, avoid refined and concentrated sugar sources such as soda, candy, pastries, and syrup, as well as sweetened fruit juices and even dried fruit. These cause your body to secrete the hormone insulin that, when combined with activity, may lead to symptoms of **rebound hypoglycemia** such as shakiness, fatigue, and lack of muscle coordination.[16]

Orange juice, dairy products with fat (skim milk is okay), chocolate, and peanut butter cause most people's bodies to secrete thick mucus throughout the digestive tract as soon as they touch the tongue. This response serves to protect mucosal linings from developing sores as acidic orange juice passes from the mouth down the food chute (**esophagus**) and helps dairy products, chocolate, and peanut butter be properly broken down for digestion. Thick mucus is bothersome when singing and can provoke breaks in phonation and excessive throat clearing. To help prevent thick mucus from interfering with your singing, avoid these substances at least two hours prior to performing.

Classical singers are trained to breathe in a way that involves a lot of diaphragm and abdominal muscle engagement. The diaphragm lowering on inhalation (**diaphragmatic displacement**) puts pressure on a full stomach and, when coupled with the postexhalation release of contracted abdominal muscles, can easily jostle stomach contents and disrupt the digestion process. Acid regurgitation and burping may occur. If you have a tendency to burp frequently, you may benefit by eating more slowly, ingesting smaller meals, and allowing at least one and one-half hours for digesting small meals before singing. Frequent burping is often a sign of reflux, a common diagnosis among classical singers, and should be evaluated by a physician.

Singers who burp often may benefit by avoiding foods that

- are very acidic and irritate the stomach, such as fried foods, fatty meats, pizza, salsa and other tomato-based products, onions, garlic, cabbage, pepper, pickles, chilies, mustard, high-**osmolality** juices (orange, pineapple, apple, grape) and wine, carbonated beverages, and spicy foods.
- cause the stomach to overproduce acid in digestion, such as high-fat dairy products (ice cream), sherbet, nuts, high-fat/fried foods, gelatin, malted milk, calcium supplements, alcohol, carbonated beverages, and caffeine.
- relax the stomach valve (**lower esophageal sphincter [LES]**), allowing acid to splash up the esophagus, such as mint (including peppermint and spearmint), chocolate, nuts, fried foods, fatty foods (including fatty meats), and alcohol. (See 5.10 Reflux and Heartburn.)

---

[16] University of California at Berkeley, ed., *The New Wellness Encyclopedia,* 98–101.

Note: Mint, peppermint especially, contains the **phytochemical** menthol that relaxes the smooth muscle of the stomach **sphincter,** thus easing stomach discomfort. Restaurant owners often use this trick by providing mints at the door so that patrons will take one on the way out and leave with nice breath, and without feeling overstuffed!

Lucy I. Spirling and Ian R. Daniels. "Peppermint: More Than Just an After-Dinner Mint." *The Journal of the Royal Society for the Promotion of Health* 121 (March 2001): 62–63. doi:10.1177/146642400112100113. Accessed August 14, 2011.

Note: Prepulcid, pronounced "preh-PUL-sid," is a medication once prescribed to stop reflux by narrowing the esophagus and tightening its lower sphincter. It frequently caused heart attacks, however, and was discontinued. Today there are no drugs that help a weak lower esophageal sphincter, only drugs that inhibit acid production or help neutralize the acid. However, high-protein foods that are lean, such as lean meat, have been shown to actually help keep the LES constricted.

Columbus Dietetic Association. *Manual of Clinical Dietetics* (Columbus, OH: Old Trail Printing, 1991), 236–240.

3.5 BODY MOVEMENT

Because singing is anaerobic exercise, it doesn't do much to help your overall physical fitness.

Aerobic exercise is important to add to your daily practice regimen. An aerobic workout will not only keep you looking and feeling healthier but also make your heart stronger, enhance your blood circulation, help to keep you at an optimal weight, and build your overall physical stamina so that you don't feel out of breath when you move and sing.

Note: It is very difficult to maintain the same volume when you're running out of breath. Some people will talk or sing until they run out of breath and have to induce muscular tension in the larynx to maintain enough subglottal pressure to finish. Over time such vocal tension can become habitual and problematic. (See 10.15 Muscular Tension Dysphonia.)

Many singers, especially those in musical theater, are often called upon to exhibit intense levels of aerobic exertion while singing on stage. As a result, they tend to develop excellent cardiovascular capabilities and their breath for singing becomes less affected by the physical demands.

The physical demands and stressful aspects of vocal performance can decrease the ability of the immune system to fight off infections. Establishing routines that increase general well-being is crucial to create and maintain a health singing voice. Just by walking a minimum of twenty to thirty minutes at a consistent but comfortable pace every day, you may find that you have more energy and cognitive sharpness.

Proper physical movement and conditioning can also help to reduce stress. Eurhythmics, Alexander technique, Feldenkrais, yoga, and dance are some recommended types of singer-appropriate body movement that visibly contribute to stage presence and poise. Power lifting is not recommended as it requires strenuous Valsalva maneuvers, which can overtax laryngeal musculature and the vocal mechanism itself. If you do lift, be sure to continue breathing throughout exertion to avoid holding your breath.

3.6 VOCAL MAINTENANCE

Water is every singer's best friend. We drink it to ward off sickness, promote thin mucus, and moisten dry throats. In fact, we guzzle away, but how much water is enough? And does that amount include soup, juice, and other liquids? The appropriate amount of water intake will vary for each of us depending on our sizes, our activity levels (including the amount of singing or talking we're doing), and the climates in which we live. Taking in too much water can actually be toxic for the body (**hyponatremia**), but it is difficult to reach this overly hydrated state. If you don't like water, you can concentrate on consuming an equivalent amount with other nondiuretic liquids and high-water-content foods such as salad veggies, fruits, soups, and even yogurt. Keep in mind, however, that your body pees out what it doesn't need, and liquids that are combined with ingredients your body can't use will lead to a little loss of the water you're consuming.

Many people don't realize this, but water doesn't actually touch the vocal folds when we swallow. This means you have to wait a bit after the water enters the stomach for it to be absorbed by the body and reach the folds. Whenever you swallow, the larynx moves up and tips forward to move the vocal folds and, more importantly, move the trachea out of the way. (You wouldn't want water to enter your lungs!) This laryngeal action reveals the esophagus that sits just behind the larynx and sends the saliva, water, or food down the "right pipe," so to speak. Maybe now you're beginning to understand why you shouldn't talk with your mouth full!

The water you drink serves your vocal folds in two ways. The first is that it superficially hydrates or **lubricates** your vocal folds like lotion on skin. This lubrication has a short-term effect and is replenished by the water you drink each day. Whenever you drink a glass of water, it takes only hours for it to reach the thousands of tiny mucous glands above the vocal folds, which squeeze it out onto the epithelial surface of the vocal folds.

Note: Most of these lubricating mucous glands lie in the saccule, ventricle, and false folds. There are a sparse few on the vocal folds themselves. (See Figure 2.2e.)

You might find that your performance benefits from drinking two to three large glasses of water (or other appropriate beverage) two hours prior to performing. This last-minute hydration gives your kidneys time to process the liquid (approximately ninety minutes), your bladder time to empty (approximately thirty more minutes), and your larynx's sub-mucosal glands enough time to begin receiving the water and depositing it onto your folds before you go on stage. When the vocal folds are vibrating two hundred or three hundred times a second during singing or speaking, they need this water to create a coating of mucus that is slippery and plentiful to prevent friction. Dehydrated vocal folds, on the other hand, are covered with mucus that is tacky and thick (**viscous**), and thus produce more friction and heat with vibration. (Think of the way motor oil in a car gets thick and gummy when it needs to be replenished after too much friction and heat.) The vocal folds swell (**edema**) in response to friction and in an attempt to insulate and cool the tissues with fluid. Swollen vocal folds vibrate less efficiently, needing more breath pressure to set them into motion, especially at high pitches.[17] Singing with swollen vocal folds is very risky; all types of problems can result. (See Chapter 10, Common Pathologies and Disorders in Singers and Possible Treatments.)

Singing requires well-lubricated vocal folds. Slippery, well-hydrated lubrication helps the folds to vibrate very efficiently, and less subglottal pressure will be needed to set the folds in motion. And there's another benefit—minimizing effort for voice production decreases your risk of most vocal disorders.

This superficial lubrication, however, is only part of how water allows your instrument to function optimally. The second way water serves your folds is that it cushions vibration. Earlier we discussed the vocal folds' multilayers and touched on an important layer just below the epithelial surface of each fold. This critical layer is the superficial lamina propria, known less accurately as **Reinke's space.** Not an empty space at all, this layer contains loosely bound tissue fibers, some tiny capillaries and glands with ducts secreting mucus and **serum** that fill the layer with a gel-like fluid. Water gets distributed to the superficial lamina propria to supply the glands and ducts with enough fluid to deliver mucus and serum into the layer. The layer is potentially cushiony depending on its hydrated state. When plenty of water is consistently available, the superficial lamina propria's fluid becomes thin and plentiful and, coupled with the loose tissue, acts as a pillow that softens the impact of vocal fold vibration during phonation. This layer also allows

---

[17] Ciara Leydon, et al., "A Meta-Analysis of Outcomes of Hydration Intervention on Phonation Threshold Pressure," *Journal of Voice* 24, no. 6 (November 2010): 638.

the epithelium above to slip and slide over the denser, deeper layers below during each vibration that passes through the fold. For the voice to perform optimally, the superficial lamina propria must be well hydrated. When water availability is low, the gel is thicker and tackier, resulting in stiffer folds that vibrate and elongate less efficiently.

Although you can relubricate the outside of the folds with water within mere hours of drinking, you cannot replenish the fluid inside the superficial lamina propria as quickly. It takes a lot longer for water to be absorbed into the superficial lamina propria. Once water is absorbed by the superficial layer of the lamina propria, it becomes "bound" to a protein that already exists in the layer called glycoprotein. **Protein-bound water** is not "free" water like the lubricating water we discussed earlier. "Bound" means you cannot directly replenish it or deplete it within hours or even with the total amount of water you drink in a day. Protein-bound water is hydrated only by long-term consistent and sufficient water intake.

Remember: Vocal fold hydration is a lifestyle rather than a day-of precaution. Drinking a lot of water the day of a performance will only superficially hydrate the mouth, throat, and vocal folds.

Note: The bound water in the vocal folds' superficial lamina propria is affected by hormonal shifts and accumulates when you experience a shift in certain hormones, such as the shifts occurring with premenstrual syndrome and menopause.

Singers who sweat a lot during a performance should continue to drink water throughout the performance. Do not overindulge with water to the point of distending your stomach, however. There is no need to be overly hydrated. As mentioned earlier, too much water can be toxic and even fatal. Do not wait until you are thirsty to hydrate either. By the time you sense thirst, you have lost 1% of your body weight to dehydration. A 2% loss weakens your performance capabilities by 10% to 15%![18]

So how much *is* enough? Your body is always trying to maintain homeostasis, or maintain internal equilibrium. Water plays a big role in helping your body with this effort. For example, the body needs plenty of water to flush out anything you take in that it cannot use and plenty more to compensate when you ingest excess salt, for instance.

Note: Did you know that American urine has been called the most expensive in the entire world due to how overnourished we are? We ingest more water-soluble vitamins than our body can use and pee out the excess.

Anthony Jahn. "Vitamins and Herbal Medicines: All Good?" *Classical Singer,* December 2001, 22.

---

[18] Nancy Clark, *Sports Nutrition Guidebook*, 2nd ed. (Brookline, MA: Sports Medicine Systems, 1997), 150–151.

But the body cannot create more water; it only has the amount you give it to work with. The body distributes water based on the average amount you tend to take in. It hydrates your vital organs first. Heart and lung function are at the top of the hierarchy; your vocal folds' singing ability is not. For water to get well distributed to lesser organs, you must be well hydrated.

The key to knowing when you're hydrated lies in the color and transparency of your urine. A hydrated body consistently produces transparent urine that is very light yellow with little to no odor, as opposed to strong smelling and cloudy darker shades of yellow. It takes about thirty days of peeing consistently clear, pale, and odorless urine for the body to reprogram itself. If you are unaccustomed to taking in the amount of fluids it takes to keep your urine pale, you will pee frequently until the body adjusts at the end of the month and begins to distribute more generously throughout the body.[19] And the added bonus is that your skin's appearance will improve too! So … pee pale to sing wet!

Note: Seventy percent of your body's volume and 50% of its weight are water when adequately hydrated.

Leon Thurman et.al. "How Vocal Abilities Can Be Enhanced by Nutrition and Body Movement." In *Bodymind and Voice: Foundations of Voice Education*, ed. Leon Thurman and Graham Welch (Iowa City: National Center for Voice and Speech, 1997), 434.

Note: My voice teacher told a singer she sounded dry in her lesson. He asked if she'd been drinking enough water, and she replied that she had. Later that day, however, the girl got up to sing in studio class and while she sang, the inside of her upper lip got stuck above a tooth. Dehydration doesn't lie! You have many major and minor salivary glands on the insides of your lips. The minor glands maintain moisture in the mouth and throat, constantly secreting and replenished by your short term, day-to-day water intake.

Sweaty summers, dry winters, and high altitudes deplete your body of water and can take a toll on your vocal folds. Maintaining at least a 40% humidity level in the air where you live, especially during winter months, is helpful.[20] Humidity level indicators called hygrometers are available at most hardware stores. Humidifiers and vaporizers can correct a dry living environment. Portable mist vaporizers are available and are a good idea

---

[19] Van L. Lawrence, "Sermon on Hydration," in *Bodymind and Voice*, ed. Thurman and Welch, 430.
[20] Leon Thurman, et al., "Cornerstones of Voice Protection," in *Bodymind and Voice*, ed. Thurman and Welch, 442–449.

for travel, especially when going to higher elevations or cold climates with low humidity levels. Cool-mist humidifiers emit a cool mist through a spinning fan that wicks tiny water droplets into the air. Vaporizers emit a warm steam or vapor from boiling water. The decision to use a cool-mist or warm vaporizer is a difficult one. Research has waxed and waned on the topic. The decision is purely one of your own choosing as both have benefits and drawbacks. Cool-mist humidifiers are considered to be safer because they do not contain dangerously hot water, but they may actually make the room feel cool. Their tanks tend to be easier to clean, and cool water that sits doesn't develop bacteria and mold as quickly as warm water. Because the mist is cool, however, the wicked water includes any germs or chemicals that collect in the tank and releases these into the room as well. Vaporizers, on the other hand, may feel very warm and comforting but contain dangerously hot water that can be problematic if there are children around and also require frequent cleaning so that mold and bacteria don't develop as the warm water sits. According to voice scientist Dr. Katherine Verdolini, vaporizers are the better choice. Because water boils at a lower temperature than most chemicals, their released vapor tends to be consistently cleaner.[21] Regardless, both options need to be cleaned often with vinegar or soap and water and **sanitized** with hydrogen peroxide to reduce the transfer of bacteria and mold into the air. Filters need to be changed frequently (probably one time per month) to maintain their function.

3.7 VOCALIZING

Before a performance, a ballerina would not simply drop into the splits without a purposeful warm-up. The vocal folds contain muscles, and like any muscle, they benefit from being warmed up and stretched before intense use.[22] Vocalize with light and easy exercises before moving gradually into vocalises that involve agility and range extremities. Doing so will help you avoid unnecessary muscle inflammation and will help prevent potentially greater vocal problems such as a vocal fold **hemorrhage**. Many professional singers who perform often enough and with great regularity, however, find that they need to warm up very little. This is especially the case for professional singers during the run of a show when vocal muscles often stay warm between performances. Rather than throwing his fastest balls just before a game, a pitcher prepares to throw his best and fastest balls by focusing, limbering up his arm, and throwing nice easy pitches. In turn, a wise singer conditions for a performance months ahead of time and the night of a performance avoids

---

[21] "Tips for Professional Voice Users and Singers," Milton J. Dance Jr. Head and Neck Center at Greater Baltimore Medical Center, Copyright 2010, http://www.gbmc.org/home_voicecenter.cfm?id=1561, accessed January 16, 2011.

[22] "Aerobic Exercise: How to Warm up and Cool Down," last updated March 20, 2009, http://www.mayoclinic.com/health/exercise/SM00067.

extreme vocalization that would tax the muscles, deplete some of the superficial hydration on the epithelium, and cause swelling. Like your pre-performance snack, you will find what works best for you and what makes you feel ready for a performance without feeling overly taxed before you get started.

A runner who runs a ten-kilometer race only to sit down immediately is going to get stiff muscles. Most runners will walk around for a while and then head over to the massage tent! The same holds true when you exert yourself singing. Use voice exercises (vocalises) that are light and gentle to cool down after an intense singing session. The easy cool-down will prevent blood from pooling in the blood vessels of the vocal folds, which would weigh the folds down. A cool-down also does the laryngeal musculature a great service by preventing postexertion tightening or cramping. Avoid talking for approximately thirty minutes after an intense practice or performance. You especially want to avoid engaging in conversation with a lot of background **noise**, so beware of cast parties and postperformance receptions. In noisy crowds you may subconsciously elevate the volume of your speaking voice to carry over the background noise level (this is known as the Lombard Effect).[23,24] Such strained speech can easily damage the vocal folds especially after a taxing performance. Like a runner's leg muscles, your laryngeal musculature needs to replenish nutrients through rest. As you use your voice for long periods of time, the muscles stop contracting as well and you begin to feel fatigue and discomfort as you lose more and more muscular control. Once you stop singing and using those muscles and rest the voice, you begin to regain strength and control. When we refer to building better stamina, we are actually referring to muscles becoming more efficient at bouncing back during rest periods. But no matter how fit a person is, no one can go on contracting a muscle forever. The body needs short breaks. You need the rests written into your songs and you need the breaks between songs during a concert, a recital, or an opera to help stave off fatigue.

> Note: The sustaining of a muscular contraction is what builds up lactic acid and causes us to tire quickly. The nonlaryngeal muscles involved in singing, such as those between the ribs and the diaphragm, contract/relax/contract/relax frequently during singing and speaking. As a result, they do not build up much lactic acid during singing and thus do not tire easily.

Singers gain endurance by sticking to repertoire and roles appropriate for their voice type or **Fach**. Appropriate "menus" of repertoire are determined by the fullness of

---

[23] Étienne Lombard (1869–1920) was a French otolaryngologist who discovered that a person's voice will involuntarily get louder when speaking in a noisy environment in 1909.

[24] Étienne Lombard, "Le signe de l'élévation de la voix" ["The Sign of Voice Rise"], *Annales des Maladies de L'Oreille et du Larynx* 37, no. 2 (1911): 101–119.

accompaniment, instrumentation, tradition, and performance venue. Until you come to really know your voice and its limitations and capabilities, you'll be wise to rely on an experienced voice teacher or coach for guidance.

3.8 MOUTH BREATHING VERSUS NOSE BREATHING

Our nostrils (**nares**) are lined with nasal hair to help filter dust as we inhale. Further in, the **nasal cavities** are lined with wet mucosa and microscopic hair-like cell strands (**cilia**) to trap and wave dust particles back and down the throat to eventually be swallowed. Because air takes a less direct route to the trachea through the nose than through the mouth, nose breathing helps to warm, humidify, and cleanse the air before it reaches the vocal folds. Nasal breathing is thus preferred for general, everyday breathing. Although it hasn't be proven scientifically, mouth breathing is generally considered by voice pedagogues to be best for singing. Inhaling through the mouth just before singing allows the mouth, tongue, and **pharynx** to be optimally positioned for the onset of the particular musical phrase. Breathing through the mouth also allows for a sufficient amount of air to be taken in more quickly than breathing through the nose. Nose breathing, however, is preferred during extended rests and musical interludes, and its benefits can outweigh those of mouth breathing when you're singing in a particularly dry or cold environment.

3.9 VOCAL HAZARDS

The various activities, environments, and behaviors that make up the following sections have the *potential* to harm the voice. After a description of the risks each poses to the voice, possible damages are divided into those that can result from short-term exposure or long-term exposure.

Inhaling irritants

Whether exhaust from automobiles, smoke from cigarettes (including second-hand smoke), or steroid inhalers for asthma, inhaled irritants pass through the vocal folds and down the trachea to the lungs. Singers must especially beware of theatrical special effects such as artificial fogs (e.g., dry ice) and smokes and pyrotechnics.

Potential damage from short-term exposure: inflamed and dehydrated epithelium and respiratory tract mucosa, lessened vocal stamina, scratchy voice quality, hindered respiration, loss of upper range and expansion of lower range, allergies, reddening (**erythema**), edema of tissues surrounding vocal folds.

Potential damage from long-term exposure: thickening of the cover, precancerous growth called **leukoplakia** (see Figures 15.3b and c), enlarged capillaries, **laryngeal carcinoma** (laryngeal cancer), lung cancer, emphysema, permanent loss of range, stiffening of vocal folds.

Exposure to loud noise

A sound source in the environment starts to vibrate (like the vocal folds) and in turn vibrates tiny particles in the air. These vibrating air particles travel through space toward your ears at 340 meters per second. The external ear (pinna) funnels the vibrating air particles into the ear canal where they strike the tympanic membrane (ear drum). The tympanic membrane delivers the vibrations to the inner ear via the three bones in the middle ear. The vibrations enter the inner ear where tiny, hairlike cilia cells pick up these vibrations, analyze them, and send them on to the brain for interpretation. When sound becomes too loud, these tiny hair cells can become damaged, on a temporary or permanent basis.[25] Once permanent damage has been done, *these hair cells die and cannot be regenerated.* There is no treatment that fully corrects damage done to hearing. The National Institute of Occupational Safety and Health (NIOSH) recommends that exposure to sound levels of eighty-five **decibels (dB)** not exceed eight hours without the use of hearing protection. Further, NIOSH recommends that for every 3-dB increase in sound level, exposure time should be cut in half to avoid hearing loss. (See Table 3.9a.) Exposure to extremely high-level noise can cause permanent hearing damage in a very short period of time. Be cautious of noise hazards and use earplugs in dangerous environments. Both commercially produced and custom-molded (more effective, but pricier) Etymotic® Musicians Earplugs® filter out dangerous decibel levels without compromising the quality and blend of sounds. These are especially helpful for long performance rehearsals. Purchasing a personal noise dosimeter (decibel meter) will allow you to check your surroundings as needed.[26] Tables 3.9a and 3.9b provide two handy guides: The first depicts the maximum length of time you should be exposed to different decibel levels listed with common noises to help you estimate loudness without a dosimeter. The second lists instruments and their respective decibel ranges to compare and measure permissible exposure with the noise chart.

---

[25] Scott McCoy compares the damage of high-**amplitude** sound on these ciliated cells to heavy furniture compacting and crushing the microfibers in carpet. The compression can temporarily inhibit or completely stop their ability to pick up a sound's vibrations and send the information to the brain. McCoy, *Your Voice,* 155.

[26] Michael Stewart, PhD, CCC-A, Professor of Audiology in the Department of Communication Disorders, Central Michigan University, e-mail message to author, October 26, 2010.

TABLE 3.9a
NOISE DECIBELS

Continuous dB	Permissible Exposure Time	Noise
40–60 dB	Any	Conversational speech
75 dB	Any	Washing machine
85 dB	8 hr	Busy city traffic
88 dB	4 hr	Gas mower, hair dryer
91 dB	2 hr	
94 dB	1 hr	
97 dB	30 min	MP3 player, tractor
100 dB	15 min	
103 dB	7.5 min	
106 dB	3.75 min	Leaf blower, rock con-
109 dB	<2 min	cert, chainsaw
112 dB	~1 min	
115 dB	~30 sec	

Information adapted from "Decibel Exposure Guidelines." Dangerous Decibels. Last updated 2011. Accessed January 27, 2011. http://www.dangerousdecibels.org/research/information-center/decibel-exposure-time-guidelines.

TABLE 3.9b
INSTRUMENT DECIBELS

Decibel Range	Instrument
75–83 dB	Bass
84–92 dB	Cello
90–92 dB	Xylophone
80–94 dB	Oboe
84–103 dB	Violin
92–103 dB	Clarinet
90–106 dB	French horn
85–111 dB	Flute
95–112 dB	Piccolo
85–114 dB	Trombone

Folprechtova, A., and O. Miksovska. "The acoustic conditions in a symphony orchestra." *Pracov Lek* 28 (1978): 1–2. Adapted from Sataloff, Robert T., Joseph Sataloff, and Caren J. Sokolow. "Hearing Loss in Musicians." In *Occupational Hearing Loss*, 3rd ed., edited by Robert Thayer Sataloff and Joseph Sataloff, 722. Boca Raton: CRC Press, 2006.

> Note: High school and university musicians and conductors are exposed to high decibel levels frequently, during rehearsals and performances. Be aware that these rehearsal and performance levels are not subject to regulations by either Occupational Safety and Health Administration (OSHA) or National Institute of Occupational Safety and Health (NIOSH).
>
> ---
>
> Vanessa L Miller, Michael Stewart, and Mark Lehman. "Noise and Hearing Loss in Musicians." *Medical Problems of Performing Artists,* December 2007, 163.

Potential damage from short-term exposure: ringing in the ear (tinnitus[27]), short-term hearing loss.

Potential damage from long-term exposure: permanent hearing loss that can make it difficult to self-monitor the voice.

Traveling by airplane or car

The air on a plane is recycled and dry, easily spreading germs and dehydrating vocal folds. As a general rule, the body will lose one cup (eight ounces) of water for every hour of flight. Cars blowing heat or air conditioning pose similar threats. Additionally, the constant **pink noise** produced by both planes and vehicles aggravates the ears and encourages vocal fatigue when trying to project to the person sitting next to you.

Potential damage from short-term exposure: dehydration, inflamed vocal folds, less than twenty-four-hour hearing loss and ringing, contraction of upper respiratory infection or other contagious illness.

Potential damage from long-term exposure: permanent hearing loss and/or tinnitus.

Vocal distortion—not glottal fry

We feel there is some confusion in the literature between glottal fry and a vocally distorted sound combined with pitch that some also refer to as glottal fry. We feel traditional descriptions of glottal fry are too simplistic and we have taken the liberty to further define glottal fry to offer some clarification on the topic. This new information is based on our opinion and not discussed in voice literature.

Glottal fry is a crackling sound that the vocal folds produce when vibrating their slowest. Glottal fry vibrations are irregular, making it impossible to track a **frequency** and detect

---

[27] More than two hundred medications and chemicals, including antibiotics and nonsteroidal medications (i.e., ibuprofin and aspirin), can cause tinnitus and even hearing loss. For more information on ototoxicity, see Barbara Cone, et al., "Ototoxic Medications (Medication Effects)," *American Speech-Language-Hearing Association,* last modified 2011, http://www.asha.org/public/hearing/Ototoxic-Medications, accessed January 27, 2011.

pitch. To create glottal fry, the false folds partially approximate, the true folds adduct completely, the body of the true folds relaxes, and the true vocal fold cover is also relaxed, flaccid, and floppy. A little air passes slowly between the true folds, and this "crackly" fry is created. To experience glottal fry, hold your breath and then allow just a little, almost no, air to escape between the folds, and let a crackly sound come through. (The false folds will begin completely contracted shut when you start a glottal fry from a breath-holding position but then relax a bit for the true folds to produce a glottal fry.) Fry is commonly used by children when pretending to be a growling lion or imitating a grizzly bear. Many voice teachers use glottal fry as a tool to relax the larynx, increase awareness of the **soft palate,** and access low notes in the chest register. This pitchless sound is produced with a very relaxed vocal mechanism and is unlikely to result in vocal damage.[28] (See **glottal fry** in 15.3 Vocabulary.)

When a glottal fry–like sound occurs *with pitch,* however, it *can* be vocally fatiguing and potentially harmful. This combination of two distinct sounds—the creaky glottal fry–like sound and a distinct pitch—is sometimes casually referred to as glottal fry. Because glottal fry is pitchless, however, this use of the term is not accurate. Crackly pitched phonation is produced in a very different manner: the thyroarytenoid muscles engage, the false folds compress inward, and subglottal pressure increases. While this increased activity and pressure may not be harmful in a very low pitch range and at low levels of loudness, it can be harmful if an attempt is made to carry it into the higher range. We'd like to call this combination "vocal distortion" to distinguish it from glottal fry. You can experience distortion by starting with a true pitchless glottal fry and then trying to maintain this as you add and raise pitch. Some country, pop, rock, and heavy metal singers use vocal distortion to create their vocal effects (just listen to funk singer Betty Davis or Britney Spears in "Oops! ... I Did It Again"). The degree of damage that distortion may cause depends on a number of factors including how loud the overall production is, the amount of breath pressure being pushed from under the folds, and the pitch. While talking, especially when tired or in our lower range, many of us habitually drop our voices at the ends of sentences into this gravelly voice. While this is not considered very dangerous, higher pitches, louder sounds, and higher breath pressure can set up a condition that is more hazardous.

Glottal fry has a bad reputation, perhaps because vocal distortion resembles fry and can be harmful. It is important to distinguish between these two variations of crackly voices. Remember, a pitchless and relaxed crackle is a true glottal fry, harmless and perhaps even useful. Two distinct sounds (fry plus a pitched sound) create vocal distortion, which is potentially damaging and should be avoided. The damages listed here are associated with vocal distortion and not glottal fry.

Potential damage from short-term exposure: vocal fatigue, laryngeal tension, erythema, edema, **polyp.**

Potential damage from long-term exposure: **nodules, contact ulcers, granuloma.**

---

[28] Michael Blomgren et al. "Acoustic, Aerodynamic, Physiologic, and Perceptual Properties of Modal and Vocal Fry Registers," *Journal of Acoustical Society of America* 103, no. 5 (May 1998): 2649.

Yelling, talking over noise, animated phonation

Vocal fold **pathology** such as a polyp or nodules in a well-trained singer is usually due to **vocal abuse** or a **vocal misuse** of the speaking voice and not necessarily the singing voice. Teaching, playing with your kids, being known as the loudest at a party, owning a dog—all of these place your vocal folds at a higher risk of being injured. Yelling, using animated phonation (e.g., loudly vocalizing a sneeze, glottal fry, speaking while inhaling, making animated character voices), and talking over noise are common culprits.

Potential damage from short-term exposure: erythema, edema, vocal fatigue, **vocal onset** delays, pitch breaks, polyp.

Potential damage from long-term exposure: loss of upper range and expansion of lower range, **hoarseness**, nodules, **varix**, hemorrhage, contact ulcers, granuloma, **diplophonia, aphonia, muscle tension dysphonia.**

Note: Rather than yelling, use hand claps, buy an amplification system for your classroom, and draw people's attention by speaking quietly and at an arm's length, also known as **confidential speech.**

Speaking pitch too low

Many people pitch their voices lower than what is natural. Disc jockeys and professional speakers are often advised to speak in a deeper voice to sound calm and make them easier to listen to. Women especially may find themselves lowering their voices to be taken more seriously. With time, this habit wears on the vocal folds.

Potential damage from short-term exposure: vocal fatigue, edema.

Potential damage from long-term exposure: nodules, polyp, contact ulcers, granuloma.

Note: A **speech-language pathologist (SLP)** can help you find your optimal speaking range so that you can speak with freedom and ease and therefore not tire. There used to be a rule of thumb that your voice should live at the pitch found a fourth above your lowest note, but this belief is outdated. Although extensive scientific research hasn't been done, it is our belief that there is no one optimal frequency or pitch. We feel that just as your singing voice has a **tessitura**—five or so neighboring pitches in which the voice likes to "live"—your speaking voice has a tessitura as well. The pitches used when you spontaneously laugh or say "mm-hmm," or those that resonate loudest when you hum from high to low with your ears plugged, tend to sit in your best speaking tessitura. Your optimal speaking pitches will feel comfortable and will likely lie around pitches that sound appropriate for your gender and age.

Loud whispering (stage whispers)

Whispering is vocalizing without vibration. It's achieved by approximating the vocal folds just enough to narrow the glottis, but not close enough to vibrate. Contrary to popular belief among singers and some voice clinicians, gentle whispering in moderation is not likely to harm the voice. Nor will the flow of air cause superficial drying, because the air passing through the glottis is hydrated from the lungs. Trying to project a whisper should be avoided, however. Very loud whispering can be superficially drying to the folds because so much air is used for speech that more frequent inhalations are needed. Additionally, the louder the whisper, the closer the folds are held together and the greater the air pressure builds below the narrow opening. For very loud whispering, the **anterior** portion of the folds close, but the **interarytenoideus** muscles have not drawn the arytenoids together to completely adduct the folds, so a posterior **glottal gap** remains. This posterior gap gives the glottis a narrowed "Y" appearance. You force air through this small posterior opening in order to whisper loudly. When you're vocally tired or hoarse, the pressure this forced air puts on the folds poses more risk than speaking quietly. If you're unsure how to whisper without constriction, you're better off using "confidential speech" or being silent and writing what you need to say.

Potential damage from short-term exposure: vocal fatigue, laryngeal muscular strain, edema, erythema, vocal onset delays.
Potential damage from long-term exposure: muscle tension dysphonia, loss of range.

Phone talk

Because of the phone's close vicinity to the mouth when you speak, you will generally tend to drop your pitch and let your voice slip into a crackly, distorted sound. (See Vocal Distortion—Not Glottal Fry in 3.9 Vocal Hazards.) Such lazy speech prevents the vocal folds from vibrating efficiently and causes the voice to tire more easily. Cocking the head to support a phone on your shoulder constricts neck musculature, compromises laryngeal posture, alters resonating spaces, tilts the linear air column, and impedes airflow. Try to stay conscientious of sitting up and using sufficient breath to support a clear, easy voice when talking on the phone. Avoid cradling the phone when speaking, and consider purchasing a hands-free phone to allow you more flexibility.

Potential damage from short-term exposure: vocal fatigue, erythema, edema, vocal onset delays.
Potential damage from long-term exposure: nodules.

Hard glottal onsets

While talking, it is normal and not a vocal health risk to use glottal onsets for words beginning with a vowel (e.g., "Ohio," "Uh oh"). These onsets require the false folds and the true folds to fleetingly adduct and be blown open with a burst of air. However, if the folds are held very tightly closed so that vibratory **onset** must be forced with a grunt-like sound, the onset is considered to be a hard glottal onset. If this excessively hard onset is produced often, the tension and force may wear on the vocal fold tissues. Hard glottal onsets are similar to, but not as severe as, clearing the throat.

Potential damage from short-term exposure: vocal fatigue, laryngeal tension, erythema, edema.

Potential damage from long-term exposure: nodules.

Throat clearing

Throat clearing aggressively slams the vocal folds together. It is generally a voluntary action and you would be wise to avoid it whenever possible. If you must clear, clear gently with nonvocalized, soft puffs of air, or even better, try a drink of water instead.

Clearing the throat in an effort to get rid of a tickle or mucus is self-defeating, because with every grinding adduction the folds swell and more mucus is produced to protect the folds from further harsh impact. The production of added mucus further instigates throat clearing and the problem is exacerbated.

Potential damage from short-term exposure: erythema, edema.

Potential damage from long-term exposure: hoarseness due to thickening of the epithelium, nodules, contact ulcers, granuloma, hemorrhage.

Coughing

Coughing is generally an involuntary response, triggered when a foreign substance touches close to the vocal folds. Often it's unavoidable. Because a cough violently adducts the vocal folds, banging them together and instigating a vicious and ineffective cycle, substitute a drink of water or gentle nonvocalized throat clear whenever possible (see earlier). If you have a cold, a cough suppressant may offer relief.

Potential damage from short-term exposure: erythema, edema, hemorrhage, polyp.

Potential damage from long-term exposure: contact ulcers, granuloma, nodules.

> Note: **Bowing** can occur following an illness or vocal fold **trauma.** We have seen patients with bowed vocal folds accompanying severe coughing. Whether the bowing occurs directly from the prolonged coughing trauma or whether the illness caused vocal fold weakness is not certain.

Suppressing a sneeze

Suppressing a sneeze is risky. The suppression creates a strong Valsalva and can strain the laryngeal mechanism to the point of hemorrhage, dislocated arytenoid, or pulled cricothyroid muscle (microtears in the muscle). Although less dangerous than sneeze suppression, sneezing with a hard vocalized onset slams the folds together and can result in vocal trauma. Try to release sneezes without tensing the throat or vocalizing. One good option is to release the sneeze on an unvoiced "ch" sound.

Potential damage from short-term exposure: edema, erythema, mild **dysphonia**, hemorrhage, polyp, pulled cricothyroid muscle (i.e., microtears in muscle fibers).
Potential damage from long-term exposure: hemorrhage, polyp, **cyst**, dysphonia.

> Note: Vocal fold cysts are associated with vocal fold traumas. Suppressing a sneeze can be traumatic to the vocal folds. Although we've never actually had a patient come in with a cyst after suppressing a sneeze, we include cyst here as a possible consequence.

Highly emotional crying

Highly emotional crying may engage thoracic fixation to such a degree that **supraglottal** musculature constricts and bears down on the larynx. On the other hand, a puppy-like whimper or soft whine can actually decrease laryngeal strain.

Potential damage from short-term exposure: laryngeal muscular strain, dryness, erythema, edema, vocal onset delays, pitch breaks, polyp.
Potential damage from long-term exposure: dysphonia, nodules.

Throwing up

Any regurgitation or vomit (**emesis**) involves stomach acid burning the esophagus and larynx to some degree. **Chronic** regurgitation may lead to the development of a chronic cough. (See 5.10 Reflux and Heartburn.) Habitual regurgitation (such as bulimia) often leads to a chronic **laryngitis**.

Potential damage from short-term exposure: edema, erythema, vocal fatigue, vocal onset delays, mild dysphonia.
Potential damage from long-term exposure: varix, hemorrhage, deepening pitch, dysphonia, laryngeal **lesion**(s), laryngeal scar tissue, contact ulcers, granuloma, discoloration of and loss of dental enamel,[29] laryngeal and/or esophageal cancer.

High doses of vitamin C (ascorbic acid)

In efforts to avoid getting sick, some singers may take large amounts of vitamin C to flush their system. Vitamin C is a diuretic, and although small doses may prove beneficial to well-being, large amounts can be very drying.

---

[29] Cosmetic alteration only; however, cosmesis concerns performers.

Potential damage from short-term exposure: dehydration.
Potential damage from long-term exposure: acidic urine.

Unsanitary humidifying

Cool-mist humidifiers and warm vaporizers can emit soothing mists for vocalists and can help to humidify a dry room, but their tanks provide perfect breeding grounds for molds, bacteria, and other pollutants to develop. Tanks should be sanitized regularly and filters replaced to ensure their effectiveness. Exposure to molds, bacteria, and other pollutants released from dirty tanks can have an adverse effect on the voice.

Potential damage from short-term exposure: none.
Potential damage from long-term exposure: allergies, oral fungal infection, respiratory illness, weakened respiratory function, vocal fold edema.

Gargling

If used regularly, a voiceless gargle with saline can reduce the number of colds and sinus infections that you get. However, gargling with mouthwash or salt water can be orally drying if used more than once a day. Beware of adding too much salt to a saline gargle as well. A saline solution typically consists of one teaspoon of salt per half cup of warm water. Excessive salt in water creates a solution that will leave salt behind after you spit, drawing out the mouth's moisture. Beware also of gargling anything with alcohol. Listerine® has a 10% alcohol content and can be especially irritating to the mouth. Use a gum-sensitive mouthwash for more frequent use and follow each gargling session with a cup of water to reduce superficial dryness. Because gargled solutions don't touch the vocal folds and are not swallowed and ingested, they do not dehydrate at the vocal fold level. Actually, they stimulate mucus to be secreted onto the vocal folds. Gargling may provide minimal medicinal benefits for some bacterial infections by superficially disinfecting the oropharyngeal cavity. Be sure to keep your gargle voiceless to conserve the vocal folds when they're inflamed.

Potential damage from short-term exposure: dryness, burning sensation.
Potential damage from long-term exposure: sores on mouth and tongue.

Prolonged voice rest

Complete voice rest (no phonation whatsoever) lasting longer than two weeks can do more harm than good for the voice. The vocal folds will actually weaken with prolonged periods of rest. After **phonosurgery**, complete voice rest lasting longer than one week is counterproductive in most patients.[30]

---

[30] Charles N. Ford, "Phonosurgery," in *Vocal Arts Medicine: The Care and Prevention of Professional Voice Disorders*, ed. Michael S. Benninger (New York: Thieme Medical Publishers, 1994), 354.

Potential damage from short-term exposure: none.

Potential damage from long-term exposure: muscle weakening (**atrophy**) causing bowing, vocal fatigue, and limited vocal range- especially loss of high notes.

Lifting heavy weights

Optimum phonation conditions occur when the body is in a relaxed and flexible state. Heavy weight lifting requires intense contraction of the vocal folds to trap a lot of air in the lungs to execute a Valsalva necessary for the exercise to achieve intense thoracic pressure.

The internal pressure created to lift something very heavy tends to also forcefully contract and tense upper chest and neck muscles to the point that the larynx is nearly immobilized. Subglottal pressure is then often released in a highly strained vocalization.

Potential damage from short-term exposure: laryngeal muscular strain, vocal fatigue, erythema, edema, vocal onset delays, hemorrhage, polyp.

Potential damage from long-term exposure: impeded laryngeal vertical movement, less flexibility, nodules, contact ulcers, granuloma.

> Note: It is also very important not to do any form of exercise with a full stomach, including water, as it can exacerbate reflux.

Singing without warming up

(See 3.7 Vocalizing.)

Singing on swollen vocal folds

> Note: Because frequency is directly proportional to the mass and weight of the vocal folds, you'll have to lengthen and push more to achieve the same pitch when the vocal folds are swollen.

Swelling means that more fluid has accumulated in tissues than what normally exists. Swelling in the vocal folds is brought on by irritation (e.g., reflux, allergies, or the common cold), a vocal abuse or misuse (e.g., hard coughing, yelling), and behavioral abuse (e.g., dehydration, smoking). Hormonal shifts (e.g., premenstrual syndrome [**PMS**], menopause) cause the bound water in the vocal folds' superficial lamina propria to accumulate as well. Swollen vocal folds are thicker, heavier, and stiffer, making them harder to control during phonation. More effort is needed to produce sound, often resulting in excessive tension and pushing the instrument beyond its capabilities.

Potential damage from short-term exposure: increased erythema and edema, vocal onset delays, vocal fatigue, laryngeal muscular strain, prolonged hoarseness, difficulty controlling voice, pitch breaks.

Potential damage from long-term exposure: **acute nodules**, varix, hemorrhage, polyp.

Singing with a sore throat

The larynx as a whole has very few pain receptors.[31] The vocal folds have *none*! When you have a sore throat, you are actually feeling the inflammation of the pharyngeal walls, not the vocal folds themselves. However, if the visible portion of your throat is red and irritated, the vocal folds likely are too. (See **pharyngitis** in 15.3 Vocabulary.) When the vocal folds are inflamed due to irritation or trauma, they usually have enlarged blood vessels. Blood is heavier than other bodily fluids, and an abundance in the folds' tiny hair-like capillaries will make singing difficult and the vocal folds more prone to hemorrhage.

Potential damage from short-term exposure: (See Singing on Swollen Vocal Folds in 3.9 Vocal Hazards.)

Potential damage from long-term exposure: (See Singing on Swollen Vocal Folds in 3.9 Vocal Hazards.)

3.10 VOCAL MYTHS

MYTH: Drink a lot of water the day of a performance

(See 3.6 Vocal Maintenance.)

MYTH: Diuretics will decrease vocal fold swelling

Diuretics will not reduce vocal fold swelling, whether the swelling is due to inflammation or a hormonal shift. When the vocal folds swell, the fluid that accumulates is in the superficial layer of the vocal folds. This fluid is *bound* by protein and cannot be affected by diuretics. (See 3.6 Vocal Maintenance.) Diuretics pull free water out of the body. As a result, diuretic pills, such as the water pill, are often taken to help eliminate bloat, but they can dehydrate you as they pull unbound free water out of your body. Keep in mind that the

---

[31] "The internal branches of the SLN supply sensory reception only for the laryngeal mucosa that is immediately above the vocal fold level and for some muscles of the larynx. The left and right recurrent laryngeal nerves … supply sensory reception for the laryngeal mucosa that is immediately below the vocal fold level, and for some muscles of the larynx." Leon Thurman, et al., "What Your Larynx Does When Vocal Sounds are Created," in *Bodymind and Voice*, ed. Thurman and Welch, 186.

fluid on and in the vocal fold epithelium is unbound free water, so diuretics *will* deplete this layer, leaving the folds less elastic and vulnerable to trauma or nodule development.

MYTH: Drinking ice water will help vocal fold swelling

It's a myth that drinking ice water after a strenuous warm-up will bring down vocal fold swelling.

Imagine your knee or eyelid is swollen. To bring the swelling down at all, ice must be held on it directly for at least ten minutes. It is impossible for the cold water to touch the vocal folds, let alone be kept near them for any length of time. Once swallowed, water passes around and behind the larynx and down the esophagus, never touching the vocal folds, and only touching the remote vicinity for a split second. Whether hot or cold, any liquid ingested will be brought to body temperature by the time it reaches the stomach and usually by the time it reaches the level of the larynx. Because the body almost immediately alters the temperature of anything that enters it, and because the time the water spends in proximity to the **laryngeal vestibule** is so fleeting, drinking ice water cannot bring down vocal fold swelling.

MYTH: Don't drink water with ice in it

Sucking or chewing on a piece of ice can, after a while, temporarily cramp the tongue's musculature and make some articulation difficult, but whether or not you should drink cold beverages is your personal preference. Research has not yet been done, but in our experience, icy beverages will not cramp up laryngeal musculature. Swallowed water never touches the vocal folds and cold water is brought to body temperature too quickly to have any cramping effect on laryngeal musculature. However, some people do feel better when they drink cold liquids, whereas others feel warm liquids are more soothing. The mucous glands in the larynx are under neurologic control, and every person has a different response to the exposures. Some may produce a thinner and more protective coating for the vocal cords with cold water and others with warm. The drink itself never touches the vocal cords and therefore can only affect them through the stimulation of the sensory receptors, which then cause a reactive production of lubricating mucus to be deposited onto the surface of the vocal cords.

MYTH: Cold fluids are absorbed more quickly than warm fluids

Contrary to popular belief, drinking cold water does not stimulate nerve receptors to absorb the water more quickly into your system. Warm and cold fluids are absorbed by the body at the same rate. Don't forget that everything that is ingested reaches body temperature (98.6°F) by the time it's in your stomach sitting, waiting to be absorbed. Temperature tends to play a role in your *consumption*, however. When you drink liquids at the temperature you prefer, you tend to drink more. Research has found that liquid is consumed in greater quantities between 50°F and 59°F.

MYTH: Gargle with olive oil and vinegar. Honey soothes the voice.

First, remember that throat is not synonymous with vocal folds and anything you gargle or swallow will not touch the vocal folds. There is no way to lubricate the folds directly except by inhaling steam. You can *indirectly* lubricate the folds by putting something in your mouth that makes your mouth water or produce a lot of thin mucus (e.g., hard candy, lemons, an apple—just thinking about biting into a Granny Smith can trigger salivation!). This digestive response will stimulate glands in the laryngeal saccule to squeeze thin (**serous**) mucus onto the tops of the folds. That said, the vinegar in an oil–vinegar mixture will stimulate a serous mucus response. The oil may act as a **lubricant** and form a very temporary film in the mouth and throat, as will honey. Glycerin encourages thin mucous production and has a demulcent effect too. Gimmicky dry-mouth cures such as "Clear Voice"® and "Entertainer's Secret"® are basically prettily packaged glycerin sprays. Some red licorice and gummy candy contain glycerin, and a little piece placed under the tongue or inside your cheek is a much cheaper way to keep your mouth from getting too dry on stage. Beware, however, of their laxative effect if eaten in large quantities! Other natural substances such as marshmallow root, licorice root, slippery elm, aloe vera, and pectin are said to have soothing demulcent effects on the throat but have yet to be well researched. Coating the throat for a significant length of time is not easy. The body's digestive response is triggered as soon as something touches the tongue and all the mucus-producing glands (not just salivary glands) are stimulated to wash everything that is ingested down to the stomach.

> Note: Be careful; use natural remedies in moderation. They, like prescription medications, can have strong adverse side effects.

MYTH: Gatorade® is the best way to hydrate singers

Gatorade® is designed to replenish bodily fluid and electrolytes lost specifically with sweat (sodium, potassium, chloride, iron, magnesium). Sodium is the primary electrolyte lost with perspiration. The sodium and water combination in Gatorade is ideal to help the body quickly replace and trap fluids after a two-hour high-sweat performance. Water will usually suffice and is preferred after a high-sweat performance that lasts less than two hours, however.[31] The many ingredients in Gatorade make it an inefficient

---

[31] http://nutritioncaremanual.org.proxy2.cl.msu.edu/content.cfm?ncm_content_id=92181, accessed October 12, 2010.

choice for general day-to-day hydration. Because your body excretes anything it doesn't need, drinking Gatorade just to stay hydrated on a daily basis will not serve you as well as water. Your body will need to use some of its fluid to flush out whatever is superfluous, unnecessarily pulling water out of your system.

MYTH: Drinking alcohol can improve performance by decreasing performance anxiety

Many performers grow dependent on alcohol to help them cope with the high stress of a performance career. Although alcohol can decrease performance anxiety, it relaxes the entire body, including every muscle involved in controlling the vocal mechanism. As a result, mental and muscular acuity needed for performing are decreased. Performers may experience weakened breath support, less vocal control, and difficulty enunciating clearly. Alcohol is also a strong diuretic, pulling water out of the body and dehydrating the system.

MYTH: Smoking makes the singing voice sexier

Smoking does cause vocal fold changes, which can, in early stages, make the voice sound sexy. Early on, the smoke dries out the true vocal folds' epithelium and the mucosal surface of the false folds and the chemicals irritate the tissues, causing some edema and erythema. Over time, however, continuous smoking causes the epithelium and superficial lamina propria of the vocal folds to dry out, thicken, and lose elasticity, eventually causing a loss of range, chronic hoarseness, and a permanent lowering of pitch. (See 10.8 Polypoid Corditis.) More importantly, the significant health risks outweigh the potential benefits of the sexy sound. The tar inhaled while smoking coats the lungs, making them less porous and stiffer, until breathing becomes very shallow and difficult. The biggest health concern, however, is the potential life-threatening development of lung, laryngeal, or mouth (including lips, tongue, and palate) cancer. Studies have shown that on average, adult cigarette smokers die fourteen years earlier than nonsmokers.[32] Moreover, the chemotherapy and radiation often used to combat cancer can scar salivary glands, leading to chronic dryness, as well as permanently decrease lung and vocal fold tissue elasticity, altering voice quality and weakening breath support.

---

[32] Centers for Disease Control and Prevention, "Annual Smoking-Attributable Mortality, Years of Potential Life Lost, and Economic Costs—United States, 1995–1999," *Morbidity and Mortality Weekly Report* 51, no. 14 (2002): 300–303, http://www.cdc.gov/mmwr/preview/mmwrhtml/mm5114a2.html, accessed July 24, 2011.

4

Troubleshooting

THIS CHAPTER IS not meant to diagnose or replace a visit to the doctor. It provides a quick way for you to navigate this book to meet personal needs and may be helpful to reference before visiting a physician regarding these symptoms. The areas to which you're directed in the book are designed to help you better understand and convey your symptoms, identify *possible* diagnoses, and discuss care options.

Some of the **disorders** that follow are not covered extensively in this book and are marked with an asterisk (*). Additionally, some of these marked disorders can certainly cause more significant symptoms before they cause the vocal issues listed.

- Nothing hurts, but you notice that the vocal folds are not functioning smoothly while singing.
  (See 5.3 Dehydration, 5.5 Premenstrual Syndrome, and 5.10 Reflux and Heartburn.)
- It feels as though there's a lump or mucus in your throat that won't go away. You cough but can't seem to clear your throat.
  (See 5.10 Reflux and Heartburn, 10.5 Vocal Fold Nodules, 10.6 Vocal Fold Cyst, 10.7 Vocal Fold Polyp, and 10.11 Laryngeal Granuloma.)
- It hurts to swallow (**odynophagia**).
  (See 5.10 Reflux and Heartburn, 10.11 Laryngeal Granuloma, 10.12 Laryngeal Contact Ulcers, and 15.3 Vocabulary: ***hyperthyroidism**, ***hypothyroidism**, ***laryngeal carcinoma**, ***pharyngitis**, and ***tonsillitis**.)

- It hurts to speak (**odynophonia**).
  (See 5.9 Arthritis, 10.2 Laryngitis, 10.11 Laryngeal Granuloma, 10.12 Laryngeal Contact Ulcers, 10.15 Muscle Tension Dysphonia, and 10.17 Arytenoid Dislocation.)
- You have difficulty warming up your voice, wake up coughing, wake up with difficulty swallowing or an acidic taste in your mouth, often have bad breath, frequently burp, have a dry cough, experience tightness in your throat or upper chest, have experienced a loss of upper range or prolonged warm-up, or vomit after eating.
  (See 5.10 Reflux and Heartburn.)
- Your voice tires as the day progresses; you have difficulty initiating phonation/vocal onset delays.
  (See Speaking Pitch Too Low in 3.9 Vocal Hazards, 5.3 Dehydration, 5.10 Reflux and Heartburn, 10.5 Vocal Fold Nodules, 10.6 Vocal Fold Cyst, and 10.7 Vocal Fold Polyp.)
- Your voice itches or tickles while vocalizing, eyes burn, and urine is dark yellow.
  (See 5.2 Allergies and 5.3 Dehydration.)
- You have difficulty phonating at all; your voice is unpredictable, hoarse, and accompanied by a constant raw or tickling sensation in the throat and urge to clear the throat.
  (See 10.2 Laryngitis.)
- Your throat and mouth are constantly dry; phonation tends to be difficult to initiate and often triggers coughing.
  (See 10.18 Laryngeal Sicca.)

5

Indirect Culprits

THE VARIOUS PHYSICAL states, disorders, and conditions listed in this chapter do not fit into one neat category. What they do have in common, however, is that none is directly related to the voice, but all tend to involve physical changes that have the potential to adversely affect the vocal mechanism.

5.1 ASTHMA

Effect on vocal mechanism: Asthma is a complicating factor for singers. The smooth muscles of bronchi, and their tiny alveoli (air sacs), narrow with overcontraction and inflammation. Wheezing is the result of air forced in and out of the channels' compressed spaces. Remember that the lungs are the driving force for the voice. If airflow is decreased, vocal stamina is decreased. As the airflow from the lungs decreases, the vocal folds must contract harder to build up the amount of subglottal pressure needed to start vibration and maintain volume. Laryngeal and neck muscles will tense in an effort to maintain harder vocal fold contraction. When the vocal folds must work so hard just to phonate, they lose some of the fine muscle and motor control capabilities attained with easy, efficient singing. Because asthmatics have decreased airflow from the lungs, they have to take more breaths while singing. This is less of a problem when the asthma is under control. Inhalers may help prevent asthma attacks, but they have their own negative side effects on the voice. Any inhaler can cause a change in the voice. The inhaled powder or aerosol must pass through the vocal folds to reach the lungs. As the medication (also called "inhaled corticosteroid" or "IHS") passes through the larynx, it can cause irritation and swelling of the vocal epithelium and change the vibration characteristics. Steroid inhalers are commonly used to control asthma and cause hoarseness in up to 55% of patients using the medication.[1-4] This hoarseness is most often due to swelling but can also be the result of a fungal infection. The use of inhaled steroids can cause a yeast or fungal infection in the mouth (also commonly known as thrush), on the back of the tongue, and on the vocal folds. This is due to overgrowth of *Candida albicans*. *Candida* and other fungal infections can be treated with medication but have a tendency to come back with continued use of inhaled steroids or oral steroids and oral antibiotics.

Remedy: As a rule, any singer with asthma should consult a pulmonologist, as pulmonologists are the experts in managing asthma. Be sure to discuss your asthma medications with a pulmonologist. Some inhalers are better tolerated than others. Powder inhalers are more likely to cause fungal infections, because they tend to deposit more powder on the folds than in the lungs. Steroid inhalers that only activate when they reach the lungs cause less vocal fold irritation. There are *oral* medications that are helpful for asthmatics and can decrease your dependence on inhalers.

If you are an asthmatic and develop voice changes, have your vocal folds examined by an **otolaryngologist.** A laryngeal *Candida* infection will need to be treated with fluconazole (Diflucan®). **Oral *Candida*** or thrush is usually treated with a nystatin mouthwash.

Note: Because what you swallow or gargle doesn't touch the vocal folds, a nystatin mouthwash will not eliminate *Candida* in the larynx.

Finally, because allergies are a common trigger for asthma, it is also important to see an allergist, who can test you for allergies and discuss with you how to best control them.

5.2 ALLERGIES

Effect on vocal mechanism: Physical responses to allergens vary. Allergies tend to cause the vocal fold cover and the mucosa of the entire resonating tract, from larynx to nasal

---

[1] D. J. Clark and B. J. Lipworth, "Adrenal Suppression With Chronic Dosing of Fluticasone Propionate Compared With Budesonide in Adult Asthmatic Patients," *Thorax* 52 (1997): 55–58.

[2] L. Fabbri et al., "Comparison of Fluticasone Propionate With Beclomethasone Disproportionate in Moderate to Severe Asthma Treated for One Year," *Thorax* 48 (1993): 817–823.

[3] S. M. Harding, "The Human Pharmacology of Fluticasone Propionate," *Respiratory Medicine* 84, Suppl. A (1990): 25–29.

[4] J. G. Ayres et al., "High Dose Fluticasone Propionate, 1 mg Daily, Versus Fluticasone Propionate, 2 mg Daily, or Budesonide, 1.6 mg Daily, in Patients With Chronic Severe Asthma," *European Respiratory Journal* 8 (1995): 579–586.

cavity, to become edematous and erythematic. Singing relies significantly on feel and, because vocal fold swelling alters the "feel" of singing, singing becomes difficult to monitor. The swelling at the vocal fold level can be enough to cause your voice to have a hoarse sound and may be severe enough to mimic laryngitis. Dampened sound **intensity** from congested resonating cavities (nose and sinuses) will further compound this sensation change. Your body will probably produce more viscous mucus as it attempts to "protect" tissues from the irritating allergen. Be forewarned: swollen vocal folds are vulnerable and using your instrument in a less than optimal state can lead you to compensate and strain. Remember, a compromised vocal mechanism is at a greater risk of vocal fold lesion.

Remedy: Get a good allergy evaluation. An allergist will test your allergic response to various allergens and identify specific things you should avoid. Request that an intradermal test be done if possible. Many allergists only do scratch tests and, according to the Asthma and Allergy Foundation of America, a scratch test alone can miss up to 10% of allergens and tend to not be as accurate as intradermal tests. Request specific allergens of interest to be tested (e.g., foods, grasses, dust, and animal dander). If you travel a lot as a singer, consider getting tested specifically for the environments in which you'll be performing. The allergist can also assist you in finding effective treatment. Remember to explain that you are a singer and need to avoid medications that are drying.

If your allergies include grass, dust, pollen, and molds (these are very common), then it may be beneficial to reduce the vulnerability of the vocal mechanism by wearing a pollen mask when mowing grass, house cleaning, or changing home air filters in heating or cooling systems. It is beneficial to change air filters monthly and to use a humidifier in the winter. (See Unsanitary Humidifying in 3.9 Vocal Hazards.)

To optimize the condition of your voice during an allergic reaction, sleep with the head of your bed raised to improve sinus drainage. Lying flat allows sinus mucus to pool in the maxillary sinus and back of the throat, irritating mucosal linings and creating moist wet areas that bacteria love. Mucus pooling primes you for a sinus infection. Avoid hard vocalized sneezing by putting the tension of the sneeze into a nonvoiced "ch" sound against the front teeth. Drink warm water or herbal tea with lemon (a lemon's acidity will thin viscous mucus), have your laryngologist prescribe a **mucolytic,** or purchase the over-the-counter **expectorant guaifenesin**. When conditions require taking further action, singers should opt for allergy shots and topical steroid sprays rather than inhalers and antihistamines. Inhalers irritate the vocal folds, and antihistamines dry out the vocal tract.

Note: Guaifenesin is most effective taken by itself and can be purchased over the counter as Mucinex®.

Note: Environmental allergies can be hereditary, so if your parents are allergic to mold, mildew, animal dander, pollen, or dust mites, you are likely to be also. Knowing your family's allergies and symptoms can be helpful.

5.3 DEHYDRATION

Effect on vocal mechanism: Dehydration at the vocal fold level is serious because dry folds are unprotected folds and are therefore susceptible to injury. A depleted superficial layer of the lamina propria diminishes the folds' cover wave and decreases the folds' cushion, leading to vocal fatigue and swelling. Repeatedly speaking and/or singing with swollen folds can lead to nodules, a cyst, or a polyp.

Remedy: Hydrate to the point of consistently "peeing pale." Water is the best choice for hydration, but it doesn't have to be the only fluid option. Steam inhalation and mucus-thinning medication can be very helpful when performing in a dry environment. Taking a mucolytic such as Mucinex® or an expectorant such as guaifenesin with water one-half hour prior to singing will help keep your folds lubricated through a performance (up to six hours). Stay away from medications that are drying prior to a performance. (See 3.6 Vocal Maintenance and Chapter 11, Vocally Hazardous Drugs.)

Note: Some humidifiers and steamers now come with tubes that can be hooked up alongside microphones. They emit a small steady dose of moisture to help the speaker's or singer's mouth from getting dry.

5.4 OBESITY

Effect on vocal mechanism: Upper body weight gain puts more pressure on the digestive tract. This pressure can force stomach acid to leak back up into the esophagus and even propel acid high enough to reach the laryngeal area. Because stomach acid is irritating to tissues outside the stomach, it can easily cause erythema and edema when regurgitated and lead to hoarseness if it regurgitates up to the larynx. (See 5.10 Reflux and Heartburn.)

The weight of a big belly can inhibit the diaphragm's ability to lower on contraction, making breath support and control more difficult. Likewise, excess upper body fat can make costal breathing more effortful. Fat can also build up in the throat, in front of the epiglottis, around the false folds, and in the tissue to the side of each true fold (though not in the true folds themselves), inhibiting vocal fold movement. Dampened resonance created by smaller resonating cavities with fattier softer walls can dull the brilliance of a voice.

The body generally works harder and fatigues more quickly when it's overweight. Overweight singers may lack the stamina required for today's performance demands. Even in opera, where the focus is on the voice and the stereotype has long been hefty singers who "park and bark" on stage, directors look for singers who dance and move with ease while singing beautifully.

Remedy: Your optimal body fat level depends on your sex, age, and heredity. Medical professionals advise that you lose weight if you weigh more than 20% over your recommended body weight. Stay away from foods that further aggravate reflux and focus on eating a low-fat diet that is high in fruits, vegetables, and whole grains. (See 5.10 Reflux and Heartburn.) Get plenty of exercise and try to match the amount of food you take in to the energy you put out.

5.5 PREMENSTRUAL SYNDROME

Effect on vocal mechanism: What causes premenstrual syndrome (**PMS**) is not well understood. Why some women get it and others not at all remains a mystery. Every woman has her own ratio of estrogen to progesterone hormones produced by the **endocrine** system in her body. Her endocrine system cyclically produces a lot of these hormones to bring on ovulation and then less to bring on a period. Some women's ratio tends to shift as the production of these hormones declines to trigger the period. This shift in the ratio of estrogen to progesterone is what triggers PMS symptoms. For some women the shift in their ratio of estrogen to progesterone is enough to cause debilitating symptoms. Others may sometimes experience a slight shift or none at all. Stress, depression, poor diet, and allergies can factor into this shift.

The larynx is greatly affected by hormonal shifts. Voice changes are associated with thyroid disorders and other endocrine diseases. Voice changes also occur with the hormonal shifts of puberty and may be experienced during pregnancy and menopause, as well as menstruation.

A French laryngologist and his gynecologist wife paired up to research the way the menstrual cycle affects the voice. They found that four to five days before menstruation, roughly 33% of women suffer from premenstrual *vocal* syndrome.[5] They actually took Pap smears and vocal fold smears in thirty-eight women during the ovulation and premenstrual stages of their cycles. Under the microscope, the smears revealed that the tissues looked similar at the cellular level and changed similarly at both points of the cycle![6] The vaginal walls, the vocal folds, and most of the larynx are lined with nonkeratinizing stratified squamous cell epithelium. This lining changes depending on the types and amounts

---

[5] Jean Abitbol, Patrick Abitbol, and Beatrice Abitbol, "Sex Hormones and the Female Voice," *Journal of Voice* 13, no. 3 (September 1999): 424–446.

[6] Jean Abitbol et al., "Does a Hormonal Vocal Cord Cycle Exist in Women? Study of Vocal Premenstrual Syndrome in Voice Performers by Videostroboscopy-Glottography and Cytology on 38 Women," *Journal of Voice* 3, no. 2 (1989): 157–162.

of hormones it receives. Progesterone, which is present after ovulation and before the period, as well as higher levels of estrogen, can cause the body's tissues to retain water and produce a bloated feeling in some women. Not only can this effect extend to the tissues of the larynx, including the vocal fold's superficial lamina propria, but also these hormonal shifts can increase the amount of water in red blood cells, thinning the blood and raising the chances of hemorrhaging, as well as weighing down the folds and impeding efficient vibration. (See 3.6 Vocal Maintenance and 10.1 Laryngeal Edema and Erythema.)

Because PMS affects some women more than others, vocal fold changes vary between individuals. Some females notice minimal changes, whereas others have significant difficulty with singing. Perceived side effects may include hoarseness, sluggish laryngeal movement, uncertainty of pitch, loss of high range and power, and vocal fatigue due to more effortful singing. Singers with strong cramps may find engaging abdominal breath support for singing too painful and thus vocal stamina will be less. In some cases, straining or compromising technique to sing with an affected mechanism can lead to the development of vocal fold lesions or hemorrhage. Many voice teachers are often able to audibly discern premenstrual characteristics in the sounds of their students' voices. Research methods so far, however, have been able to show only minimal measurable differences (predominantly in **jitter**).[7] Perhaps just as acoustic measures cannot measure the beauty or feel of a tone, they may not yet be sensitive enough to accurately detect the degree of vocal changes during PMS.

Remedy: To reduce your risk of hemorrhaging, avoid taking aspirin and aspirin substitutes when you're going to be using your voice a lot. **Acetaminophen** (Tylenol®) or a cyclooxygenase-2 (COX-2) inhibitor such as Celebrex® will not thin the blood and are your drugs of choice for cramps and headaches, but beware of the dulled sensation these create while singing. Because these drugs mask pain, you will have a decreased sense of when your voice is feeling tired or pushed. The premenstrual period is also associated with increased nausea and throwing up after **general anesthesia**. Avoid scheduling any surgery during this portion of your cycle.

Note: Some European opera houses have granted female singers grace days in their contracts to refrain from singing around the onset of menstruation!

V. Lacina. "Der Einfluss der Menstruation auf die Stimme der Sängerinnen." *Folia Phoniatrica* 20 (1968): 13–24. Cited in Filipa Lã and Jane W. Davidson. "Investigating the Relationship Between Sexual Hormones and Female Western Classical Singing." *Research Studies in Music Education* 24 (June 2005): 77. doi :10.1177/1321103X050240010601.

---

[7] Sung Won Chae et al., "Clinical Analysis of Voice Change as a Parameter of Premenstrual Syndrome," *Journal of Voice* 15, no. 2 (June 2001): 278–283.

5.6 PREGNANCY

Effect on the vocal mechanism: Your vocal folds may swell as estrogen and progesterone levels significantly increase your blood volume up to 55%, as well as trigger your body to retain salt and water.[8] You may even feel winded in the first trimester before you even begin to show. Your body demands more oxygen when it's pregnant, and the increase of hormones, progesterone in particular, stimulates the respiratory area of your brain. This stimulation can leave you feeling out of shape just from walking across a room. Respiration is also impeded as the fetus grows. Most women experience shortness of breath from the second trimester on as the diaphragm has less room to lower, limiting the lungs' ability to fill on inhalation. The decrease in diaphragmatic motion also makes it more difficult to sustain held pitches and support long phrases. As breath support decreases, your vocal folds will be forced to sustain a harder contraction on adduction to build up the subglottal air pressure needed to project the voice. This added effort can cause the vocal folds to fatigue quickly. Over an extended period of time such effortful singing can lead to muscle tension dysphonia and vocal fold damage. (See 10.15 Muscle Tension Dysphonia.) You may have difficulty maintaining abdominal support if you experience belly button discomfort, round ligament pain, and/or abdominal cramping as tissues stretch and organs are pressed to relocate to accommodate the expanding uterus. Even the degree to which your abdomen distends in the last trimester can hinder normal abdominal muscle function. You're more likely to experience reflux triggered by the extra weight put on during pregnancy. (See 5.4 Obesity.) Additionally, your baby's growth pushes the diaphragm upward, and the fluid-filled stomach is caught in between. This pressure on the stomach

Anecdote: I (Dr. Rachael Gates, primary author) was already experiencing round ligament pain, belly button pain, and feeling out of breath toward the end of my first trimester. Staying mindful of my limitations, I continued to teach privately and perform occasionally well into my third trimester. I found that as my baby began to grow inside of me and my lungs' vital capacity began to decrease, the effect on my breath felt much like that of the corsets I had to wear under costumes in period operas! While I was limited in the amount of breath I could take in, I had a heightened sense of resisting collapse on exhalation, and the sensation of leaning on the breath (appoggio) was powerfully distinct. Perhaps your voice teacher has tied a scarf snugly around your ribs, then asked that you resist allowing the scarf to slacken as you sing a long phrase. This common exercise is used to help singers identify what it means to lean on the breath. Having something to resist while staying expanded is a helpful tool in learning how to use breath support, and being pregnant gave me an extreme awareness of this.

---

[8] Michael S. Benninger, "Medical Disorders in the Vocal Artist," in *Vocal Arts Medicine: The Care and Prevention of Professional Voice Disorders*, ed. Michael S. Benninger (New York: Thieme Medical Publishers, 1994), 208.

Note: Although there is no scientific research on this yet, anecdotal evidence suggests that due to their familiarity with the low pressure that thoracic-abdominal inhalation puts on their abdominal organs—including the uterus—classically trained females may push more efficiently and have shorter labors than other women!

tends to also aggravate reflux, which can in turn lead to vocal erythema, edema, and hoarseness. Whether from constant effortful voice use or reflux that reaches the laryngeal area, vocal fold inflammation leaves the mechanism more vulnerable to hemorrhage during vocal exertion brought on by labor and delivery.

Remedy: Little can be done for the shortness of breath that often accompanies fetal growth. Recognize your voice's limitations under such conditions and avoid voice injury by not compromising your technique to attain a desired sound that might be impossible due to symptoms out of your control. (See 5.10 Reflux and Heartburn.) You may want to be especially conservative with practice and performing in the third trimester especially, because this is the time when physical limitations, discomfort, and fatigue are often greatest.

5.7 MENOPAUSE

Effect on the vocal mechanism: Some women will enter **perimenopause** as early as the late thirties, while most will start to notice symptoms closer to age fifty. Because menopause tends to be hereditary, you will likely begin to experience symptoms at the same age your mom did.

As you enter perimenopause, you may experience hot flashes, mood swings, irritability, and irregular periods due to the fluctuation in hormones. Scheduling performances around periods will be difficult during this time. Your vocal folds' epithelium begins to thicken during perimenopause, and the fluid in the superficial lamina propria layer thickens as well. Although your voice may not yet start to sound different, the thickenings will likely cause your voice to feel different. You'll likely feel that you have less control of the voice and need to work harder to produce the same sound.

Vocal fold tissues eventually lose elastic and collagenous fibers, making it difficult to sufficiently elongate for your highest notes.

Once you are in menopause, you no longer get a period. Progesterone levels have dropped to zero, androgen levels drop by 50%, and estrogen levels have dropped as well. Body temperature and mood become consistent again. Your voice is permanently lower (likely 10 to 15 **Hz**), with a decreased upper range. Your voice is likely less flexible and less capable of smooth register shifts between chest voice and head voice.

Remedy: Consider hormone replacement therapy issued by a knowledgeable endocrinologist. You may relieve symptoms and minimize vocal changes by beginning estrogen supplementation as soon as **premenopause** begins. Normal estrogen levels are reported as a range and an individual may be on the high or low side of normal. Standard dosages of hormone replacement therapy may put you back into a normal range, but it may not be your normal level. It's therefore a good idea to have your obstetrician/gynecologist test your mid-cycle peak estrogen and progesterone blood levels before you reach menopause. By her late twenties or early thirties, a woman's singing voice has likely matured, making these good pre-menopausal ages for hormonal baseline testing. Getting exact levels is not critical, but don't wait until your late thirties when it's possible that you'll already be entering perimenopause. You want to get close to premenopausal levels for potential future hormone replacement therapy so that the therapy will be more effective at bringing you back to your normal levels.

Note: Androgen supplementation is not advised for female singers. Even small amounts can cause a permanent change in timbre, vocal instability, and lowering of the voice.

5.8 OLD AGE

Effect on vocal mechanism: It is normal for our bodies to weaken and stiffen with advanced age. When the natural aging process affects the larynx, it is called **presbylarynx** or presbyla-rynges. Presbylarynx is made visibly evident when the muscles inside the vocal folds, like all muscles in the body, begin to atrophy and cause **bilateral** bowing of the vocal folds, but there are other signs, too. (See 10.9 Bowing.) Women's estrogen and progesterone levels fall and androgen levels rise as they near menopause, and their voices steadily drop 10 to 15 **Hz**. Men's voices get deeper until their early fifties and then begin to get higher as their testosterone levels drop. The vocal folds lose elasticity and thin with the decrease in collagen. Eventually, a wobble may develop in the voice as nerves atrophy and their firing slows down. Ligaments weaken and joints typically lose some of their range of motion with age, affecting the arytenoids that swivel to bring the vocal folds together and apart. At around seventy years old, the muscles involved in inhalation, exhalation, and breath support begin to lose power as well, and sustaining pitches and projecting the voice become increasingly difficult.

Remedy: Consistent healthy use of the voice slows the natural atrophy process of all muscles involved with vocal production. Our instruments generally age at the same rate that our bodies age, and while there are hereditary factors involved in the aging process, the old phrase "use it or lose it" still applies. Regular vocal exercises (vocalises) and singing with good technique on a daily basis will keep both the singing and speaking voice strong and agile for a longer period of time. Overall physical condition is important. Routine cardiovascular and aerobic exercise such as swimming, jogging, walking, and yoga help to maintain the posture, energy level, stamina, and pulmonary (lung) function needed to sing well. Singers should never take extended periods of time away from singing after fifty years of age. If you are over fifty and take several weeks off from singing, you will have great difficulty getting back to your previous level of function. (See 5.7 Menopause.)

5.9 ARTHRITIS

Effect on vocal mechanism: The tiny joints of the larynx are similar to the other joints in the body. There are tendons, ligaments, articulating surfaces, and fluid-filled spaces involved. Injury to any of these structures can limit the joints' range of motion or cause pain with motion. As with other joints in the body, overuse or misuse can also lead to the degeneration of the laryngeal joints. The movement of the vocal folds requires fine motor control and easy resistance-free motion. Any small impediment to their motion can result in significant vocal changes.

The earliest symptoms of laryngeal arthritis are usually increased difficulty controlling the upper register, a decrease in the voice's upper range, and prolonged warm-up time. The cricoarytenoid joints and/or the cricothyroid joints may be affected. The upper register of the voice requires both arytenoids' maximum ability to rock backward over the top of the cricoid surface, to further tense the elongation of the vocal folds. If either cricoarytenoid joint is injured, its rocking motion may be limited and unable to fully extend and thin the vocal fold for high pitches. Another possibility is that the arytenoid will be able to rock backward enough to fully elongate the vocal fold's length but too much effort is required to maintain the position and high tones become unstable. Cricoarytenoid joint stiffness is similar to stiffness in one of your fingers. If a finger joint is damaged, the finger has less motion and feels stiff. With continued use the joint will "loosen" and move with greater ease. However, as the joint becomes more involved, the motion can become uncomfortable or even painful. Likewise, a cricoarytenoid joint that is stiff from injury may loosen with a prolonged warm-up period but will not withstand sustained effort.

Cricoarytenoid arthritis is not a common problem but neither is it rare. Cricothyroid arthritis is rare, but still worth mentioning. The symptoms are comparable to those described earlier. Because the movement of the cricothyroid joint elongates the folds, inflammation and stiffness in the joint make hitting high notes difficult. Arthritic laryngeal joints are most commonly found in those with rheumatoid arthritis, and rheumatoid arthritis can show up in laryngeal joints prior to other joints. If you have any of the previously mentioned symptoms, a family history of arthritis, and/or other joint pains, arthritis should be considered. Diagnosing cricoarytenoid arthritis is still often difficult. Arthritis that affects both cricoarytenoid joints will cause difficulty breathing and speaking. Advanced cricoarytenoid arthritis, on the other hand, can lead to a fixed or frozen joint and is often confused with a **vocal fold paralysis**. Physicians will listen for difficulty transitioning into a higher range and will look for a cherry red arytenoid, asymmetric swelling on an arytenoid, and improvement with an anti-inflammatory medication.[9] Clinicians will look

---

[9] W. W. Mantgomery, "Cricoarytenoid Arthritis," *Laryngoscope* 73, no. 7 (2009): 801–836.

for a decrease in the motion of one vocal fold, as well as mild vocal fold bowing or asymmetrical vibrations due to mismatched tensions placed on the vocal folds. These are fine distinctions, however, and are often only detected by a clinician with extensive experience looking at fold vibrations. Even when a thorough voice exam doesn't reveal any pathology, cricoarytenoid arthritis should still be considered if your vocal complaints are disproportionate to the physical findings and conventional **voice therapy** is not helping. Often there are not any visual characteristics other than mild swelling around the inflamed joint. For this reason, cricoarytenoid arthritis is often misdiagnosed as reflux disease because of the similar swelling both present at the back of the larynx. Reflux is a much more common vocal issue than cricoarytenoid arthritis, and usually only a lack of response to reflux therapy will suggest arthritis. A trial of arthritis medication should be done if symptoms are present and there is a lack of improvement with reflux therapy.

Remedy: The treatment of cricoarytenoid arthritis is similar to other forms of arthritis. The only difference is the tiny size of the joint involved. For acute flare-ups, immediate treatment may require a short-term high dose of a corticosteroid such as prednisone to get stiffness and swelling down. More chronic mild arthritis may respond quickly to non-steroidal anti-inflammatory medications such as over-the-counter ibuprofen or naproxen sodium. Acetaminophen (Tylenol®) and COX-2 inhibitors such as Celebrex® are safer drug choices for arthritic pain, because they won't thin the blood. You may require regular daily doses of medication or a dose only before singing. (Many runners with arthritis in the knees need medication only prior to training in order to run the distance required.) Those with advanced arthritis should be treated by an arthritis specialist, known as a rheumatologist. A rheumatologist will evaluate arthritis through blood tests and, depending on the test results and symptoms, select from numerous prescription medications that are available in various strengths for treatment.

Note: It's never too early to begin keeping a detailed file on your family's medical history. Finding out whether your relatives have had rheumatoid arthritis, lung cancer, or heart issues will raise your awareness of what you may be susceptible to so that you can live preventatively.

5.10 REFLUX AND HEARTBURN

Effect on the vocal mechanism: The esophagus leads from the throat to the stomach, and the sphincter entrance to the esophagus is located behind the larynx, just posterior to the arytenoids. The esophagus has a lower sphincter as its entrance to the stomach. Sphincters allow things to pass through one way and immediately tighten up to prevent anything from escaping. The lower esophageal sphincter (LES) allows food to enter the stomach but keeps the acid in the stomach from sloshing up the esophagus during digestion. If the stomach has produced too much acid or if the LES is weak, acid may leak into the esophagus and burn its lining. It's normal for stomach acid to enter the esophagus from time to time.[10] Occasional reflux is called physiologic reflux and is not likely to cause any damage.

However, there is another type of reflux called **laryngopharyngeal reflux** (**LPR**) in which acid not only leaks into the esophagus but also gets sloshed all the way up to the vocal fold and pharynx area. Even one LPR event is considered abnormal. Laryngeal tissue is not equipped as esophageal tissue is to handle stomach acid. Stomach acid is especially irritating to laryngeal tissue, and even one episode of acid regurgitating up to the laryngeal level can cause enough erythema, edema, and increased mucus to interfere with vocal production. Those affected often experience a need to clear the throat, post-nasal drip, a lump feeling in the throat, difficulty warming up, quick vocal fatigue, and hoarseness. Reflux may cause a burning sensation in the chest that is commonly called heartburn, although the sensation has nothing to do with the heart. Reflux can also trigger or aggravate asthma. Singers, especially classical singers, are prone to LPR due to the vigorous diaphragm and abdominal movement involved in singing. Because LPR causes heartburn sensations in only about half the people it affects, however, it's not always easy to detect. LPR is also known as silent reflux because it tends to occur at night while you're lying asleep and may not stimulate laryngeal tissues enough to disrupt a heavy sleeper.

The seriousness of reflux is determined by how often reflux events occur, how acidic the reflux gastric acid is, and how long it sits in the esophagus. You could have reflux that stays in the esophagus for a long time and not cause damage if the pH is not too low (typically a pH under 4 is considered acidic enough to cause some problems[11]). A tiny bit of reflux that is really acidic is worse than a lot of reflux that isn't as acidic. A gastroenterologist will use all these factors to determine whether a reflux problem is a chronic disease called **gastroesophageal reflux disease** (**GERD**). If left untreated, GERD can erode the lining of the gastrointestinal tract and cause bleeding and/or tissue changes such as peptic ulcers (gastric and duodenal ulcers), grayish-white thickening of the tissue between the arytenoids known as **pachyderma**, precancerous thickening of the vocal folds called leukoplakia (see Figures 15.3b and c), scarring, abnormal vocal fold motion called **paradoxical vocal fold movement** (**PVFM**), tracheitis/tracheobronchitis, esophageal narrowing (**stenosis**), anemia, and in rare cases cancer. You can have occasional LPR but not technically have GERD disease.

---

[10] L. F. Johnson and T. R. DeMeester, "Twenty-Four Hour pH Monitoring of the Distal Esophagus: A Quantitative Measure of Gastroesophageal Reflux," *American Journal of Gastroenterology* 62, no. 4, (1974): 325–332.

[11] Radu Tutuian and Donald O. Castell, "Gastroesophageal Reflux Monitoring: pH and Impedance," *GI Motility online* (May 2006), doi:10.1038/gimo31, accessed August 22, 2011.

Note: Heartburn, the burning sensation at the lower end of the sternum, is just one symptom of reflux. Many who have reflux do not experience heartburn. Of the patients seen at the Ohio State University Hospital Voice Clinic, we estimate that over half of the patients show evidence of reflux-related change in their larynxes and claim to not have heartburn.

Remedy: Avoid lying down after eating. Lying down tips your stomach's contents, encouraging stomach acid to leak back into the esophagus. Wait about three to four hours after eating to get into a reclining position so that gravity can help keep stomach contents down and out of the esophagus during digestion. Elevate the head of your bed four to six inches by putting bricks under the bedposts or create a wedge under the mattress. (Piling pillows under the head is not sufficient. They elevate only the neck, not the torso, and they shift around.) Decrease the pressure on the stomach by losing weight if overweight. Eat smaller meals slowly so as not to overstuff the stomach and cause the LES to relax. Avoid constipation and straining when going to the bathroom; both increase the pressure in the stomach. Refrain from bending at the waist after eating and do not exercise with a full stomach. Even the thoracic fixation involved with a very low abdominal breathing technique used especially among classical singers can aggravate reflux due to the pressure it places on the stomach. Therefore, it is not wise for those susceptible to reflux to sing on a full stomach. Even if the stomach is only filled with water, exercising, bending, and thoracic fixation can still trigger reflux. Be conservative with the amount of acid in your diet by limiting pizza, salsa and other tomato products, alcohol, caffeine, oranges, grapefruit, and other acidic fruits and juices. Stay away from things your stomach must neutralize by producing more acid, such as ibuprofen, mints, cheese, milk, and nuts. (See 3.4 Foods to Avoid and Why.) You can also avoid triggering more acid production by managing stress. If you smoke, stop. The nicotine in cigarette smoke relaxes the stomach sphincter and increases acid production as well. For occasional reflux, take over-the-counter antacids (e.g., Tums, Rolaids) when you eat problematic foods. They will neutralize your stomach acid immediately and remain effective for approximately one hour. Be careful however, as antacids can lead to mineral imbalance if taken for long periods of time! For weekly occurrences, opt for H_2 blockers (a.k.a. H_2-receptor antagonists) such as Zantac® or Pepcid®, which actually reduce the acid in your stomach. Within thirty minutes, these will block acid from being produced in your stomach, but they work best when taken intermittently and are not as effective at blocking acid when taken on a consistent basis. Reflux that occurs more often than two times a week and can't be controlled by behavior modifications, may require stronger, longer-lasting medications called proton pump inhibitors. These are available in low doses over the counter (e.g., Prilosec®, Prevacid®) or prescription strength (e.g., Prilosec®, Nexium®, Protonix®, AcipHex®, and Prevacid®). To take effect, these must be taken at the same time consistently to build up in the bloodstream and will take roughly twenty-four hours to begin controlling symptoms. (See 11.10 Gastrointestinal/Reflux Medications.)

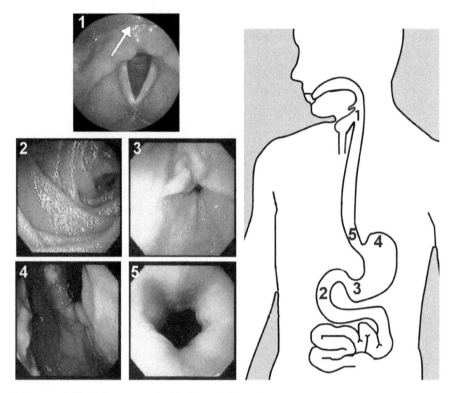

FIGURE 5.10 Upper Gastrointestinal Endoscopy
This simplified diagram exaggerates the esophagus to focus on the digestive tract (or food pathway) and path of the scope. The larynx and trachea are implied by the outline just anterior to the esophageal entrance in the neck. The numbers on the diagram are placed according to the scope's location when it captured the photos on the left. To capture the first picture, the flexible scope was inserted orally and positioned to peer down onto the vocal folds and esophageal entry. Please refer to Figures 2.2g and 2.2p for further anatomical clarification. (1–2: Entering the digestive tract via the esophagus. 3–5: Pulling the scope back out of the gastrointestinal system.) 1. Healthy vocal folds. The arrow marks esophageal inlet or entrance where the larynx meets the back pharyngeal wall. The gastrointestinal endoscope is passed into the esophagus. 2. Healthy duodenum (first section of small intestine). 3. Healthy antrum (near bottom part of stomach). 4. Retroflex view (looking up at healthy gastroesophageal junction/lower esophageal sphincter from underneath). 5. Bottom of esophagus, specifically, lower esophageal sphincter from above.

Note: Acid-reducing medications do not interfere with digestion. The stomach has more than enough acid, pepsin, and other digestive enzymes to digest food. Even if you totally removed the stomach, you could still digest food lower in the intestinal tract!

If you have chronic reflux issues, you may want to consider having an upper gastrointestinal (**GI**) endoscopy (see Figure 5.10) to determine the cause of gastric reflux and check for possible raw sores (**ulcerations**) and precancerous changes in the linings of the esophagus, stomach, and duodenum (the beginning of the small intestine).

5.11 OBSTRUCTIVE SLEEP APNEA SYNDROME

Effect on the vocal mechanism: **Sleep apnea** occurs when some part of the airway obstructs breathing during sleep. During sleep, the soft tissues of the soft palate, throat, and tongue relax and can be sucked into the airway on inhalation enough to stop breath flow. Sleep apnea generally develops from **adenoids** and **tonsils** becoming enlarged (**hypertrophy**), but people who simply have small resonating cavities are at a higher risk of airway obstruction during sleep, too. Sufferers experience laryngeal tension and sleep deficiency, leading to chronic tiredness and a low threshold for vocal fatigue. Sleep apnea can easily trigger reflux as well. As airflow is interrupted on unsuccessful attempts to inhale, a siphon is actually created and acid may get sucked back up from the stomach into the esophagus. Severe sleep apnea can strain the heart and lead to serious health problems such as heart attacks, high blood pressure, or pulmonary failure.

Remedy: Because consistent airflow pressure is needed to keep the airway open while sleeping, wearing a continuous positive airway pressure (CPAP) mask over your nose can help those with sleep apnea. The CPAP continuously feeds just enough air to keep the upper airway passages from collapsing. Losing weight can also help if you're overweight, because fat that accumulates in the resonating cavities makes them smaller and softer. Sleep on your side rather than flat on your back, the latter of which lends itself to gravity pulling the soft tissues into the airway, interrupting inhalation. Avoid drinking alcohol and taking sleep medications, as both decrease hydration and relax laryngeal musculature, making it harder for you to breathe while sleeping. If tonsils and adenoids are the culprit, an adenotonsillectomy may be the answer. (See Sleep Apnea in 12.3 Common Problems Where Surgery Could Affect the Vocal Mechanism.)

6

What Purpose Does the ENT Clinic Serve and

How Will It Serve You?

6.1 THE ENT CLINIC

An ENT (**otolaryngology**) clinic specializes in disorders of the ears (**otology**), nose (**rhinology**), and throat (**laryngology**). An otolaryngologist will treat hearing loss, nasal and sinus disorders including allergies, throat disorders such as tonsillitis, voice disorders, and numerous other disorders related to the head and neck region. Otolaryngology is considered a surgical specialty. Because otolaryngologists examine difficult-to-see areas, they will utilize state-of-the-art equipment and instrumentation to assist in the physical exam. An ENT clinic is the preferred setting for singers seeking care, because an otolaryngologist is the only type of physician with training concerning the voice.

6.2 THE VOICE SPECIALISTS

All otolaryngologists are medical doctors (MDs) who have received the same basic training regarding the ears, nose, and throat. They've completed four years of medical school and have specialized by going on to complete a five-year ear, nose, and throat residency. Few of these otolaryngology residencies, however, offer much in the "throat" category. Otolaryngology residents do perform laryngeal surgeries but are not instructed at a highly technical level. Most receive their degree without ever learning how to read laryngeal **stroboscopies** and may not even know anything about voice disorders, especially with regard to the singing voice.

Otolaryngologists may choose to go on with their education and **subspecialize** by completing a one- to two-year fellowship in a field such as neurotology and otology, rhinology, facial plastic surgery, or laryngology. Seeing an otolaryngologist who has completed a fellowship in laryngology ensures optimal care for the professional singer. A laryngologist is an otolaryngologist who has subspecialized by completing an extensive laryngology fellowship in voice disorders and phonosurgery. The laryngologist is the physician of choice for singers.

> Note: "Phonosurgeon" is the European term for laryngologist.

Most laryngologists will work in a clinic that deals specifically with voice disorders. These specialty clinics, also known as **voice clinics**, involve a team of experts specializing in the voice. The team includes speech-language pathologists and personnel to evaluate singing techniques. Ideally, a voice clinic will be affiliated with a clinical voice pedagogue. A clinical voice pedagogue is someone who has an understanding of the vocal arts and the medical and scientific aspects of the voice and is a highly trained singer. This singing health specialist is best suited for evaluating the singing voice and the subtle abnormalities that can affect the singer. She is an excellent resource when the laryngologist or speech-language pathologists are unable to identify a problem.

> Note: Certification in singing health is still new, and an official title is not yet recognized by the American Speech-Language-Hearing Association (ASHA).

The speech-language pathologist has the initials **CCC-SLP** (Certificate of Clinical Competence—speech-language pathologist) following their name. SLPs deal broadly with disorders of communication and swallowing. A minority of SLPs will specialize in voice disorders. These subspecialized SLPs feel comfortable working with singers and evaluating their vocal folds. Some speech-language pathologists are also voice pedagogues (having degrees in both music and speech pathology) and will work with singers on singing technique when health is concerned.

The role of the SLP is to assist the physician with the diagnosis and treatment of the patient. From swallowing to phonation, SLPs are trained to assess the entire vocal tract using their eyes and ears, as well as special diagnostic instruments. They do not actually make a diagnosis, but the information they obtain through case history, identification of vocal abuses or misuses, and diagnostic exams may help the physician with his decisions.[1] The SLP often works as a valuable filter between the patient and laryngologist by spending thirty minutes to an hour talking with and examining the patient and relaying assessments to the laryngologist before his ten-minute exam. The SLP is not authorized to prescribe medication. Although a laryngologist provides all medical therapy, SLPs help treat and prevent diseases of the vocal folds by performing voice therapy. You may consider an SLP a sort of physical therapist of sports medicine. When an athlete pulls a muscle, a sports medicine technician frequently helps the athlete rehabilitate. Similarly, SLPs help rehabilitate the voice. They set timetables for recovery and assess progress by performing diagnostic tests. It will be up to you to find an ENT clinic that has a laryngologist and an SLP experienced with professional singers. (See Chapter 7, A Vocalist's Guide to Finding the Right ENT.)

Lastly, voice instructors are voice specialists. These personal trainers for singers are established singers themselves. They may or may not have extensive scientific understanding of the instrument, but they definitely understand the voice from firsthand performance experience and teach with aesthetic empathy for you and your voice.

6.3 WORKING AS A TEAM

No one physician has all the answers. Beware if a physician thinks he has all the answers, especially if his solution involves an immediate recommendation for surgery. Although some voice disorders and lesions do require surgery, many do not. Surgery is always the last option for a disorder or lesion that has a chance of recovering on its own, with therapy or medication.

Your care extends beyond the larynx and requires an interdisciplinary team. You will obtain the best care through the combined efforts and knowledge of the primary care physician, laryngologist, speech-language pathologist, voice instructor, and, most importantly, yourself. Understanding your own instrument makes you a valuable member of the team in assessing, treating, and especially preventing future vocal problems.

Once you have been diagnosed with a problem, your voice instructor plays a significant role in your vocal recovery. She is expected to encourage you through the rehabilitation process and, with your approval, is welcome to attend therapy sessions, as well as view recorded examinations of your condition. Once the team agrees that you're well enough to sing, the voice instructor is responsible for gradually guiding you back into healthy singing and eventually performing.

The interdisciplinary approach is most effective when everyone's goal is to restore the vocal mechanism to its optimal health and maximal function. The goal is not a quick fix but a long-term maintenance program. However, regardless of the medical concern, the ultimate responsibility for the well-being of your voice rests with you. You must be in touch with your body and willing to take charge of your voice.

---

[1] "It is the position of ASHA that vocal tract visualization and imaging for the purpose of diagnosing and treating patients with voice, resonance/aeromechanical, or deglutition disorders is within the scope of practice of the speech language pathologist." American Speech-Language-Hearing Association (ASHA). "Vocal Tract Visualization and Imaging: Position Statement," (2004) PS2004–00121, http://www.asha.org/policy, accessed August 8, 2011. doi:10.1044/policy.

7

A Vocalist's Guide to Finding the Right ENT

7.1 WHY GO?

JUST AS YOU would go to great lengths to find the right private voice teacher, so should you seek out a voice clinic equipped with up-to-date instrumentation and well-informed medical specialists. Building a trusting relationship with a qualified laryngologist is key to any singer's good health. The specialized expertise and authority of the laryngologist offers you protection when dealing with other physicians and aids you in emergency situations. Visits to the ENT clinic should not be just about problem solving. Like any physician, laryngologists are much more effective in treating a person when they know the person inside and out. You need the laryngologist to know your lifestyle, vocal demands, and personality to reduce the sense of urgency and crisis when problems arise and to enable appropriate decision making.

To help the laryngologist know your voice, consider getting "voice headshots." That is, have photos and a video taken of your folds in their optimum condition to be kept on file at the ENT clinic. Schedule a baseline visit at the clinic when healthy, warmed up, and in good voice. Request copies for your own portfolio as well. The pictures and video of your healthy instrument can serve as a barometer for future visits, something with which to compare if and when you have problems. These copies are especially helpful for voice emergencies during travel.

7.2 WHOM TO ASK

Finding a competent laryngologist (or otolaryngologist when a laryngologist is not available) should be one of the first orders of business for a singer. Consult any of the well-informed resources listed here for recommendations.

- Laryngological associations:
  American Laryngological Rhinological and Otological Society, Inc.
     http://www.triological.org
- Opera directors/singers/voice teachers/coaches found in:
  Local opera companies
  Universities
  Conservatories
- Speech-language pathologists found in:
  Speech-pathology departments at large hospitals
  Speech and hearing departments at major universities
- Singers may also keep well informed by keeping association or membership with
  the following organizations:
  American Speech-Language-Hearing Association (ASHA)[1]
     http://www.asha.org
  National Association of Teachers of Singing, Inc. (NATS)
     http://www.nats.org
  American Choral Directors Association (ACDA)
     http://www.acdaonline.org/
  Music Teachers National Association (MTNA)
     http://www.mtna.org/
  Acoustical Society of America
     http://http://asa.aip.org/
  Voice Foundation
     http://www.voicefoundation.org/

7.3 WHAT TO ASK

Not all otolaryngologists and ENT clinics are equipped or have the expertise to work
with singers and diagnose specific problems common to singers. Otolaryngologists and
laryngologists are trained to perform surgery, but not all actually perform surgery. Some
otolaryngologists refer to themselves as laryngologists but have never done the subspecialty fellowship. It is important as a singer to ask pertinent questions to ensure quality
care. Remember, this is your instrument and not all otolaryngologists are created equal!
Request a consultation and an examination session. Use the session to gather information
about the physician and to see if your personalities are compatible. It is very important
that you feel comfortable with your doctor and he with you. Conduct an interview with
the prospective physician or his staff. Do not question the physician in a way that may be
perceived as doubting his ability to treat a singer. Doing so may offend the physician and

---

[1] ASHA is also a good source for finding a qualified SLP with singer experience.

permanently destroy the doctor–patient relationship. The following suggested questions can help you determine whether or not an otolaryngologist is well suited to your needs:

Note: You may find the answers to many of these questions on the physician's practice website or by asking the employees at the clinic.

- Are you certified by the American Board of Otolaryngology? (See **board certified** in 15.3 Vocabulary)
- Do you or anyone in the practice subspecialize in voice disorders and phonosurgery?
- Do you have specific training (e.g., a specialized intern process or fellowship) in dealing with the singing voice?
- What type of singers do you see regularly (e.g., classical, country, rock, etc.)?
- How extensive is your history treating laryngeal problems in performing artists?
- Do you perform surgery?
- Would you call your approach in treatment and surgery conservative?
- Do you have any speech-language pathologists (SLPs) and singing teachers with whom you work closely?
- Do you work closely with an SLP who specializes in voice?
- Are you an active member of any professional voice-related organizations?
  American Medical Association
  Board of Otolaryngology on Head and Neck Surgery
  American College of Surgeons
  Collegium Medicorum Theatri (CoMet)
  Laryngologic Society
  Triologic Society
  American Speech-Language-Hearing Association (ASHA)
  The Voice Foundation
  National Association of Teachers of Singing, Inc. (NATS)
  The International Association of Logopedics and Phoniatrics
- Are there publications or research papers you've written to which I could gain access and read?
- Do you personally know of a good voice teacher?

It's optimal to select an otolaryngologist who:

- has a working understanding of your singing style and is experienced treating professional singers who sing in that style,

- answers yes to all the yes or no questions listed previously,
- attends meetings and/or has presented papers for two or three of the mentioned organizations,
- offers the titles of a couple papers he's authored relating to professional voice use, and
- suggests a respected voice teacher that you may contact as a reference.

8

The First Visit and Procedure

A VISIT TO a voice clinic may include some or all of the components described in this chapter. The exact process may vary from clinic to clinic.

8.1 HOW LONG WILL IT TAKE?

First visits generally take up to two to three hours, especially if a video study is going to be performed. Allow yourself plenty of time so that you may relax and get to know the clinicians. This will help you determine whether or not you feel comfortable with their abilities and personalities. Subsequent visits may take only an hour.

8.2 WHAT THEY NEED TO KNOW ABOUT YOU AND WHY

Plan on filling out a case history sheet each time you visit the ENT clinic. Filling out the forms will require knowledge of medications (keep an updated list in your wallet) and problems, past and present, vocally related and not. Remember, anything relating to your health may affect your voice. Following is a list of case history questions you're likely to be asked. Be prepared to answer all that apply.

SYMPTOMS

Do you have any of the following symptoms?

Hoarseness	Breathiness	Vocal fatigue	Bitter/acidic taste in mouth	Loss of pitch range
Can't sing	Tickle/cough	Bad breath	Hoarse in morning mostly	
No voice at all	Heartburn	Hard to swallow	Regurgitate food	

VOICE

When did your problem begin?

How did it start? Gradually or suddenly?

Any pain at the start?

Any pain now?

What makes it better? Worse?

Do you use your voice extensively at work?

What treatments or therapy have you tried?

Which voice part do you usually sing: soprano, mezzo, alto, tenor, baritone, or bass?

Have you studied singing? Where? For how long?

What types of music do you usually sing?

BREATHING

When did your problem begin?

How did it start? Gradually or suddenly?

Do you feel short of breath?

Is this feeling exertion induced or spontaneous?

Does it occur in episodes/attacks?

How often does it occur?

What makes it better? Worse?

Do you wake up choking?

Do you have a chronic cough?

Is the cough productive or nonproductive?

Do you use inhalers? (Please specify.) Are they effective?

Do you hear wheezing when you breathe?

Is the wheezing present on inhalation, exhalation, or both?

Have you experienced any verbal, physical, emotional, or sexual abuse?

SWALLOWING

Do foods stick in your throat?

Do you tend to choke when eating?

Do any certain food consistencies give you greater difficulty than others (water, thick liquids, pudding, puree, solids, pills)?

DIET/LIFESTYLE

Do you use/have you used tobacco products? How much per day? For how long? When did you quit smoking?

Is your workplace or home smoky?

Do you drink alcohol? What kinds? How much per week?

How many cups of coffee, tea, soda, or other caffeinated beverages do you drink daily?

How many glasses of water do you drink daily?

Do you typically eat dairy, spicy, fried, and/or fatty foods? Peppermint, mint, onions, garlic, citrus fruits or juices?

Do you typically eat close to bedtime?

Any recent weight gain? When and how much?

How would you rate recent stress levels in your life—mild, moderate, or severe?

MEDICAL HISTORY

Are you allergic to topical anesthetics?

Do you have any medication, food, or environmental allergies?

Do you often have nasal congestion, sinus congestion, or postnasal drip?

List all current and recent medications you have taken regularly (prescription and over the counter).

List all previous surgeries.

Have you been diagnosed with any of the following medical conditions?

Diabetes	Cancer
Arthritis	Thyroid disease
Emphysema	Hearing loss
Multiple sclerosis	Parkinson disease
Sinusitis	Heartburn/reflux
Hernia	High blood pressure
Asthma	Heart disease
ALS	

Other conditions (stroke, pneumonia, migraines, etc.)?

The questions you answer in writing while sitting in the lobby may be asked again by the physician or other clinician during your visit. Though seemingly redundant, verbal explanations often reveal more than those you wrote down. The written forms are filed in your medical chart for future reference. Offer any previous pictures of your vocal folds so that the physician may better determine your present state. (See 7.1 Why Go?) Be honest and thorough when answering questions and offering information. Not only must you trust your laryngologist, but also he must be able to trust you. To assist in an accurate diagnosis, it's important for you to describe your problem as you experienced it, in your own words. Remember that the physician will benefit if you're also able to explain your vocal complaints in terms that are familiar for him. After all, the physician can only effectively treat you if he understands your complaint. Pay attention to how much your physician understands the singing voice. Consider using some "singer" terms to see if the physician is comfortable with the vocabulary. If you get a blank stare, this may indicate a vital communication barrier and a lack of familiarity with the singing voice. This does not mean the physician is not knowledgeable, but would suggest a lower level of experience with singers and indicate that you should look elsewhere for help.

After you leave the clinic, the laryngologist will probably dictate a summary of your visit to be kept with your chart. If your visit included a session with a speech-language pathologist (SLP), the SLP will also write up a summary to include in your chart.

8.3 INSTRUMENTS USED IN THE CLINIC

This section helps to demystify the various diagnostic instruments and equipment you might see and get to experience at a voice clinic. By understanding what they do, where they go, and why they're used, you may have no reservations with them being used on you. You might also call ahead of a visit to check whether they have a certain instrument you are interested in requesting at your exam.

The Laryngeal mirror

A tiny mirror, similar to that of a dentist, can be used to look at your folds. (See Figure 8.3a.) This procedure is called an **indirect laryngoscopy** or **mirror imaging** and is the most common approach used for viewing the vocal folds. In some patients' conditions, it may be the only exam that is required. When you have no vocal complaints and a check-up is all that is needed, a mirror exam is often sufficient if a good view is obtained. Combined with a halogen light worn on the head, the laryngeal mirror is the best method for getting an overall view of the larynx and for viewing colors of the anatomy accurately. This combination may

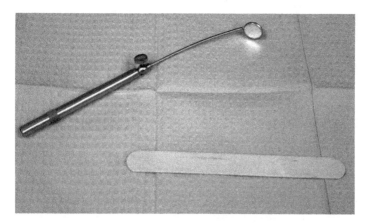

Figure 8.3a The Laryngeal Mirror With Tongue Depressor

reveal large lesions and let the clinician know whether or not the folds open and close properly, but it cannot detect vocal fold vibration and, depending on the patient's anatomy, cannot always be angled to capture the entire length of the vocal folds. Another disadvantage is that the mirror can only obtain a view of the vocal folds while you are breathing or holding a single tone and not during connected speech or singing. If you have a significant vocal complaint, a **laryngoscope** should be used to more thoroughly examine the vocal folds.

Anecdote: One physician using a mirror to examine a patient with hoarseness viewed what appeared to be a perfect pair of vocal folds. However, he was only seeing half the folds. He thought he had exposed the entire length of the folds with the mirror, but what appeared to be the anterior commissure were actually nodules! Had he positioned the mirror farther past the epiglottis, he would have seen that the meeting of the vocal folds was premature.

The Scopes

Laryngoscopes are instruments used for viewing the larynx. The types used in the clinic offer a clearer and more defined view of the vocal folds through magnification. (See Figure 8.3b.) There are two basic types of clinical scopes, flexible and rigid, and they are often attached to a video camera to allow both moving and still pictures of the larynx. A recorded examination using either of the two scopes is called a video laryngoscopy.

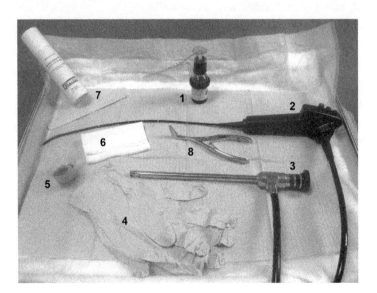

Figure 8.3b Clinical Scopes and Materials
Photo of instruments and supplies on sterile barrier cloths. Not pictured: Lubricating jelly for nasendoscopy and disinfecting solution. 1. Afrin®-lidocaine nasal anesthetic spray. 2. Flexible nasendoscope. 3. Rigid oral endoscope. 4. Sterile latex-free exam gloves. 5. Antifogging solution. 6. Gauze. 7. Benzocaine oral anesthetic spray (cherry flavor) and tongue depressor. 8. Nasal speculum.

The video exam provides a record for viewing at a later time and allows slow motion replay to improve diagnostic ability. This is especially helpful for patients with a strong gag reflex that prevents anything more than brief views to be obtained.

The **nasendoscope** is a skinny flexible scope, similar to but a little thinner than a cable TV cord, that passes into the nostril, through the nose, behind the palate, and behind the base of the tongue until the tip of the scope hangs just above the laryngeal area. This procedure, commonly called a **nasendoscopy**, is also referred to as "macro" **laryngoscopy** because it provides a view of the entire larynx and throat (pharynx). It takes about five minutes but can go on indefinitely to observe activities such as talking and singing. Unless nasal passages are obstructed or too tiny, the freedom of activity makes the nasendoscopy the preferred exam for children, as well as for evaluating singing technique. It is also the method of choice for patients with a strong gag reflex, because the scope hangs in a way that it is unlikely to touch gag-sensitive areas.

The **rigid laryngoscope** is a 20-cm-long wand that is passed orally, like the mirror, to the back of the mouth. The wand is positioned just past the tongue and just below that little dangling punching bag at the back of your mouth called the **uvula**. The end of the scope has an angled opening of usually about 70 degrees. This angle enables the examiner to peer over the back of the tongue at the laryngeal structures without touching the back pharyngeal wall. Many skilled clinicians are able to balance the wand in their hand during insertion so that it touches nothing and provokes no gagging. Of course, if the **oral cavity** is small, the scope may touch the tongue or roof of the mouth in order to obtain the best view. Even so, most people tolerate the procedure with little to no gagging. Because this procedure, commonly called an **oral endoscopy**, focuses solely on the vocal folds, it may also be referred to as "micro" laryngoscopy.

Note: You might hear or come across the terms "microlaryngoscopy" and "macrolaryngoscopy" in reference to your exam. "Macrolaryngoscopy" suggests a more holistic evaluation of the larynx and vocal tract, as is done with the flexible scope during phonation or singing. "Microlaryngoscopy" focuses in on the vocal folds and their free edges in particular. Most often, you will hear microlaryngoscopy (or microlaryngology) used to refer to the examination of the larynx that occurs in an operating room during **microlaryngeal surgery**. The exam involves peering directly down on the larynx via an operating laryngoscope using magnifying binocular lenses. (See Figures 12.5a and 13.4a.)

The rigid oral **endoscope** and a special type of nasendoscope called the Chip at the Tip (a.k.a. Chip-Tip, Chip on the Tip) Videoscope best illuminate and magnify the vocal folds and provide the clearest close-up view of the surface and free edges of the vocal folds. Both are able to evaluate slight color changes and small vocal fold lesions and are able to assess the vibration of the vocal folds. Some small voice clinics with limited funds may only have one scope. If a clinic has only one scope, the scope will likely be a nasendoscope because of its ability to view nasal passages and the entire larynx on a more "macro" level, and because of the general view and observation options this scope offers. The nasendoscope may not be the Chip at the Tip Videoscope model, however. Older nasendoscope models are **flexible fiberoptic laryngoscopes** that produce very poorly lit, low-resolution, and slightly distorted fish-eye images of the larynx. They are unable to detect all color nuances and, coupled with the distorted image, are not ideal for evaluating the vocal folds' vibrating edges.

The Electronic equipment

The images captured by both scopes are projected onto a monitor that the clinician observes throughout the procedure. (See Figure 8.3c.) The type of light in both scopes is halogen and provides the sunny brightness needed to observe accurate color, general laryngeal movement, and appearance. Halogen lighting is ideal for capturing a beautifully lit still image for your file, but it doesn't allow you to see any vibration. Because the folds vibrate 50 to 1,500 **cycles per second** (**cps**), they are too fast to observe with the naked eye. Under any constant light, the folds simply look closed and fluttery when phonating. To actually view vibration and any vibratory characteristics, the clinician needs to illuminate the vocal folds with a specially timed flashing strobe light (**xenon light**). The name for the recorded exam that uses this timed strobe light to help diagnosis is **video laryngeal stroboscopy** (**VLS**). A VLS can be performed by an otolaryngologist or an SLP with a nasendoscope or an oral endoscope and is the exam of choice for singers. Although an expensive procedure, this recorded strobe study offers the detail necessary to diagnose a singer with a voice complaint. To perform a VLS, the clinician will hand you a stethoscope-like laryngeal microphone to hold against the side of your thyroid cartilage or will strap a small microphone around your neck. Her choice will depend on whether she prefers to use the **electroglottogram** (**EGG**), which requires the microphone to be strapped to the side of your thyroid cartilage. The EGG microphone is hands-free (and may be more comfortable than you or she holding the stethoscope). It also offers more information: whereas the stethoscope picks up only how many times your folds are vibrating per second (**fundamental frequency**), the EGG displays the length of time the vocal folds are open or closed in each cycle (phase closure). (Some clinicians can gather enough phase closure information just by looking at the folds' movement on the monitor and don't always need the more accurate measurement of the EGG.) The clinician uses a foot pedal to change from halogen to strobe lighting. (See Figure 8.3c detail.) Then, by depressing the mode button with her foot, she can change the speed of the strobe's flashing from fast phase to slow phase to zero phase as needed. When the clinician needs more detail she chooses slow phase, triggering the strobe light to create an impression of slow motion vibration. The vibratory motion that is displayed on the screen is not the folds' true continuous vibratory cycle slowed down from real time. Rather, the flashing light works with the fundamental frequency detected by the stethoscope to pick up a

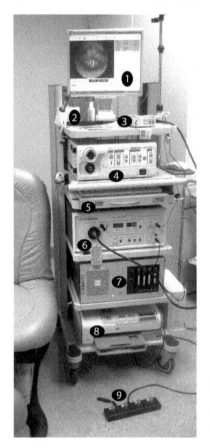

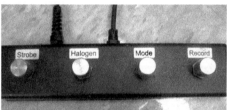

FIGURE 8.3C The Electrical Equipment (left) and Foot Control Pedal detail (right)
Left: There is no electroglottograph on the system pictured. 1. Monitor. 2. Speaker. 3. Camera body for both scopes (with image focus). 4. Video processor with Chip-Tip flexible endoscope port (xenon light only). 5. Keyboard. 6. Xenon and halogen light port. 7. Hard drives (removable for archiving exams), DVD drive, USB ports. 8. Printer. 9. Foot control pedal. Right: The strobe and halogen buttons allow switching between types of lighting whether color or movement is being assessed. The mode option allows toggling between phases of vocal fold closure. The record option is available to capture a portion of the exam at any point to be saved in the patient's file. Still pictures are also created from what is recorded.

certain ratio (i.e., "slices") of your folds' vibrations and create a slow motion picture of the vocal folds opening and closing. You will need to sing straight tone during a VLS, because vibrato has too much variation in frequency and the device will not be able to track a central frequency. This slow phase method of viewing the folds' motion relies on your vocal folds having a steady, regular (**periodic**) vibration to get a realistic simulation of vocal fold vibration.

The clinician may choose slow phase to get a good view of the lower portion of the folds as every cover wave passes from the bottom to the top of the fold. If the clinician wants to check your vibratory pattern for asymmetry, she may select fast phase. The fast phase option works the same way that slow phase does, but the simulated slowed vibration is somewhat faster.

> Note: To see vocal folds vibrate in real time requires a very high-speed camera that can image the vocal folds at such a high frequency. This technology is available but requires much memory to store the number of frames it takes to record just one exam. It also takes a very long time to play back all the frames recorded. For these reasons, high-speed imaging of vocal fold vibration won't replace stroboscopy just yet. It is, however, a valuable tool for viewing irregular vibrations in detail or for looking closely at specific aspects of vibration that require just a few frames such as onset and offset.

The zero phase button captures a picture of the vocal folds at the same point in every cycle. The shot is timed to frequency so that if phonatory patterns are regular, a consistent open or closed phase will show. In other words, as long as the sound is steady and the vibrations are periodic, the zero phase option gives the impression of a "still" image. You will need to sing straight tone for the strobe to track your frequency. Vibrato can throw off this measuring device, which relies on a consistent pitch frequency. The clinician can select the zero phase option when she wants a view of how the folds look at a specific point of every vibration (e.g., only their completely open or closed phase of each cycle, or somewhere in between) for a sustained length of time. More often, however, she uses the zero phase as a way to diagnose whether the folds have irregular (**aperiodic**) vibrations. Vocal folds with aperiodic vibratory patterns will have motion evident in the freeze picture, implying some kind of instability in producing a tone. The instability may be due to a neurological disorder (such as **spasmodic dysphonia** or an **essential tremor**) or a structural disorder (such as bowing).

Before beginning the procedure, the clinician will type your name into the computer and attach or have you hold a microphone or stethoscope against one side of your Adam's apple. She may ask that you say your name or count to ten. This allows her to observe the vocal frequency display on the monitor and ensure that it's sensing your voice. Once the procedure is over, the clinician should invite you to observe the video with her while she explains what was found. If the clinician doesn't show you the results, feel free to ask! Laryngoscopies are often recorded and saved indefinitely for future reference. Still pictures are selected from the video, printed, and filed with your chart. Request copies of photos for your own documentation and bring in a blank multimedia storage device for a copy of the exam as well. (Check in advance to find out what the clinic's recording system uses.) Making a copy of your exam can take some time and the clinic may ask you to return later to pick up your copy. They may also require you to pay a small fee for this service.

8.4 UNDERSTANDING HYGIENE IN THE CLINIC

Because the ENT clinicians are dealing with people's mouths all day long, many precautions are taken to ensure that each procedure is sanitary. The process varies from center to center. At some centers, the clinician performing the exam may simply disinfect all used instruments in Cidex® for a minimum of twenty minutes between patients and then rinse them well with water before reusing. On the other end of the spectrum, there are clinics and hospitals that have a trained staff dressed in protective clothing (i.e., paper gowns, facial masks, gloves) who do nothing but ensure that the disinfecting process of the scopes is followed rigorously. They first perform a dry leak test by hooking an endoscopic leak tester up to the scope and blowing air into the scope through a special port. A pressure gauge tests for holes along the scope's sheath. Additional staff, often nurses, may perform a second test by submerging the pressurized scope in water and checking closely for bubbles, which would also reveal any hole in the sheath. Next they soak the scopes and all procedure utensils in an enzymatic, low-foam detergent such as OptiPro® to "de-goop" the instrument of mucus. Then they submerge all instruments in a disinfecting solution such as MetriCide® OPA for twelve minutes (five minutes to kill 98% of germs and seven more minutes to kill tuberculosis, according to experts at the James Care Voice and Swallowing Disorders Clinic). Finally, the nurses rinse everything for three minutes under running water to ensure all chemicals are removed. Instruments are relaid on carts covered with sterile barrier cloths ready to be delivered for the next exam.

All clinicians must wash their hands before and after the exam. All clinicians handling equipment and examining the patient are required to wear sterile gloves. Once the gloves are on, extreme care is taken not to contaminate the scope. The clinician's hand that holds the patient's tongue in gauze during the procedure is considered contaminated and may not touch the scope or anything other than the patient's mouth. This leaves only one hand available to handle the scope and is why a floor panel of controls is used—so that the feet may adjust equipment. Once the exam is complete, all waste is deposited into a receptacle, also operated by the foot, and the sanitization process is repeated.

Note: You should inform the physician if you are allergic to latex. Many rubber examination gloves contain latex, and latex-free gloves should be available if needed.

Note: Did you know that "sterilize" and "disinfect" are not synonymous? Sterilization is a process that kills *all* living microorganisms. Disinfection is a process such as that involving alcohol or chlorine bleach that eliminates *most* harmful microorganisms, other than bacterial spores. Chemicals, radiation, or heat can be used to achieve either state.

8.5 WHAT THEY WILL DO, WHERE THEY WILL PROBE, AND WHY

The Anesthesia

Generally speaking, a laryngeal exam should include inspections of the ears, nasal passages, mouth, and throat. You will remain fully conscious throughout all these inspections and will rarely need **topical anesthetic** to counteract discomfort. Nevertheless, the clinician will most likely begin by offering to use a topical anesthetic spray in the nose or mouth, such as lidocaine, benzocaine, or **Cetacaine**®, before the throat portion of the examination. These **anesthetics** behave much like the Novocaine® used by dentists but are sprayed topically rather than administered through a needle and do not last as long. The mirror exam and the oral endoscopy are painless procedures that may require numbing only in patients prone to gagging. The nasendoscopy may cause slight discomfort in some patients, but in our experience most patients do not feel they need the anesthetic.

> Warning: Avoid eating or drinking for one hour after receiving topical anesthetic. The anesthetic reduces oral sensation, making you less coordinated while chewing and swallowing and more likely to choke.

The Exam

Depending on what is being evaluated, a typical vocal fold exam can be completed in ten minutes. The scope is typically in place only one to three of those minutes, according to the patient's comfort level.

The laryngologist begins with indirect laryngoscopy to examine the vocal folds. He will prep the mirror against fogging by running it under hot water or coating it with a blue antifogging liquid. A bright light worn on his head will be used to light the back of your throat and reflect off the mirror. He may ask you to say "aaahh" first in order to flatten your tongue and take a good look at your oral cavity, tonsils, and soft palate. Then, holding your tongue with a piece of gauze and pulling it out slightly or depressing it with a tongue depressor, the physician guides the mirror into your mouth until it is just below or against the uvula. This provides a reflected view of the anatomy behind and below the tongue. This exam requires good tongue and palatal control by the patient. Try to keep the tongue relaxed throughout the exam so that the tongue base doesn't pull back or raise, obstructing the view. If the physician feels a closer look is necessary, he will decide to use a scope or more likely have one of his SLPs perform the laryngoscopy.

> Note: The laryngologist should always scope a singer who has a voice complaint, rather than rely on a mirror, due to the complexity of singing issues.

The type of scope used for your exam will vary depending on your ability to tolerate the various procedures and what aspects of your larynx are being checked. The clinician will choose to perform a nasendoscopy if she needs to evaluate soft palate movement, breathing through the nose, talking, singing, swallowing, or moving around throughout the exam with ease. Before the clinician inserts the nasendoscope, she may gently peer into each nostril using the nasal speculum and directly spray the inner passages with a numbing solution if needed. She will lubricate the flexible nasendoscope with a water-soluble lubricating jelly, such as Surgilube®, and press the power button on the foot panel to turn on the scope's halogen light. She then will focus the camera by holding the scope's tip over the computer keypad and adjusting the picture of the letter key that appears on the monitor via the image focus button. Lastly, she will dip the tip of the nasendoscope into water that is warmer than body temperature or an antifogging solution that coats the lens so your breath doesn't fog the lens and cloud the picture.

> Note: Every patient is different, but based on our experience you may find the following hints helpful. Helpful hint #1: Before the clinician inserts the nasendoscope, determine which nostril is more open by closing off one nostril at a time and sniffing. Helpful hint #2: You may request a nasal anesthetic spray that also contains Afrin® (such as the one pictured in Figure 8.3b) in order to constrict blood vessels and widen nasal passages prior to inserting the scope. Helpful hint #3: Keep your eyes open during the exam to distract yourself from tensing up, and breathe through your nose to help open the nasal passages and gently guide the scope into the nose.

As the clinician inserts the scope into your nose, the light from the nasendoscope illuminates the inside of your nasal cavity. (See Figures 8.5a and 8.5b.) She turns to the monitor to see the image and sees three tiny passageways: the lower (inferior), middle (medial), and upper (**superior**) **meatus**. She chooses the meatus that appears the most open (often the inferior or middle tend to be a nice one-half to three-fourths inch in diameter) and passes the nasendoscope through. You'll feel a brief pressure in your nose as the scope passes between the **turbinates,** but it quickly ceases and the monitor shows that the scope has cleared the passageway and is behind the nose in the upper throat space called the **nasopharynx.** (See Figures 2.2g and 8.5c.) The clinician continues to pass the scope down into the midthroat portion of the pharynx at the back of the mouth called the **oropharynx** until the camera is looking down into the **laryngopharynx** and onto the vocal folds.

> Note: The superior meatus is tiny and rarely used to avoid pain and viewing the larynx from an odd angle. The medial meatus and inferior meatus are the clearest, most open passageways through which to feed the cord. (See Figure 8.5a.)

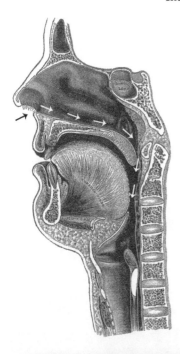

FIGURE 8.5a The Nasendoscope Route

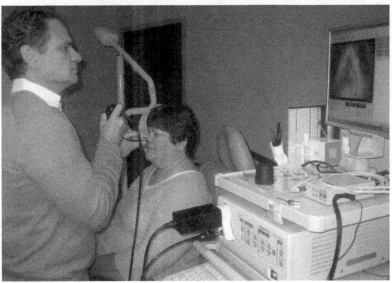

FIGURE 8.5b The Nasendoscopy

The exam may sound uncomfortable, but it really is not too bad. It may feel a little strange to have a thin cord-like scope inserted in your nose. Its stimulation to the sinuses may trigger involuntary eye watering, slight discomfort, a tickle sensation, or very rarely a minor nosebleed while passing through the nasal passage. Once the scope's camera is in place, however, you'll likely feel comfortable.

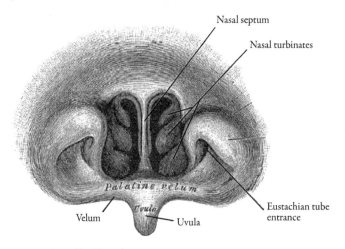

Nasal septum

Nasal turbinates

palatine velum

uvula

Velum

Uvula

Eustachian tube
entrance

FIGURE 8.5C The Nasopharynx
This is the view looking up from the back of the mouth through the velopharyngeal port behind the uvula into the nose. This is the way the dental floss and nasendoscope are passed into the oropharynx.

Note: If you were to open your mouth at this point in the exam and look in a mirror, you'd see the scope hanging just behind and below your uvula! This brings a gross memory to mind: The dental students I knew in school thought it was neat to pass one end of a piece of dental floss through a meatus in the nose by sniffing it in and swallowing, encouraging the floss to hang down at the back of the throat. They'd open their mouth and grab the other end to floss their nose!

Note: Did you know the floor of your nose is the roof of your mouth?

The clinician will want to look very closely at your vocal folds, especially if you're a singer with a vocal concern. Singers often sense minor discrepancies with their voices out of a heightened awareness they've developed for fine singing. To evaluate the more intricate details of your vocal folds, the clinician will do an oral endoscopy. Activity during this examination is limited due to the endoscope's oral interference, but the oral endoscope offers the best magnification and illumination of the vocal folds, revealing better detail of the vocal folds and surrounding laryngeal structures. The clinician will defog the tip of the oral endoscope into warm water or the antifogging solution. Then she'll power the halogen light with her foot and focus the scope's camera on the computer keypad. She will ask you to stick out your tongue and breathe through your mouth. Remind yourself to breathe through your mouth. Breathing through the mouth helps to keep your soft palate up and retracts sensitive tissue away from the scope so you can avoid gagging. Remember to relax your tongue so the clinician may hold it with a piece of gauze and pull it out slightly.

Note: The clinician will likely provide you with the following hints to help ensure that she can capture a good picture. Hint #1: Sit forward in your chair and place your feet flat on the floor. An upright posture is optimal for viewing the larynx with an oral endoscope. Hint #2: Extend your neck and chin out like a turtle in a "sniffing position" to allow the oral endoscope to capture a better view of your larynx.

As the clinician positions the wand in your mouth, by either guiding it across the tongue or balancing it between the tongue and uvula, she focuses on the monitor to be sure she is capturing the image correctly. (See Figure 8.5d.) She then uses the foot pedal to click pictures for your file. Be sure to ask the clinician or physician for a copy of your exam photos for your own record (or wallet)!

Warning: Remain still during the insertion and removal of the oral endoscope. Although it happens very rarely, sudden movement could result in a chipped tooth!

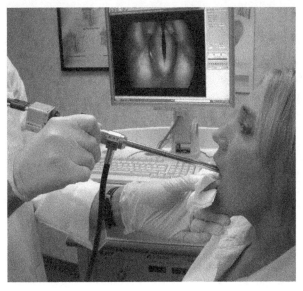

FIGURE 8.5d The Oral Endoscopy
Courtesy of Kay Pentax.

Sounds you will make and why

For a successful mirror exam, you will be asked to hold an "eeee" sound during the exam in order to view the larynx. During an oral endoscopy, the clinician will ask you to perform various tasks on vowels, much like simplified vocalises. To help her attain the most accurate evaluation of your voice, make sure you go to your exam as warmed up as your vocal condition will allow and that all sounds you make during the exam are supported. The clinician will likely begin by holding your tongue and asking you to sustain "eeee" at a comfortable pitch. Achieving a pure "eeee" sound will be impossible with your tongue held. However, your attempt to sing a pure "eeee" raises the back of the tongue up and pulls it forward, exposing the larynx more fully to the camera and bettering the clinician's chances of capturing an image of your anterior commissure. The clinician will likely depress the stroboscopy pedal with her foot to begin a VLS and look at the regularity (**periodicity**) of your vocal fold movement while sustaining the "eeee" vowel. If a lesion is present, the consistency of the lesion can often be determined by whether it moves with the folds or is so stiff that it obstructs vibration. Evaluating lesion consistency can determine if therapy might be helpful or if surgery is needed for resolution. The clinician may also ask you to sing "hee hee hee." The [h] sound is called an **aspirate onset**. The repetition of the aspirate onset allows the camera to capture vocal fold motion and how the folds come together, so the clinician can determine whether there is excessive muscular involvement, vocal fold weakness, **paresis**, and asymmetrical movement. This method is also used to clear mucus from the folds when trying to distinguish between a vocal fold lesion or thick mucus on the folds. The clinician may remove the scope and ask you to swallow or gently cough if there is still uncertainty or if there is mucus that obstructs her view. Performing a glide from the bottom of your range to the top of your range is also commonly requested. Pitch breaks in the glide indicate that the vocal folds' vibration is irregular (aperiodic) due to vocal fold edema, muscle tension, dehydration, or vocal fold stiffness. The inability to glide up may suggest a paresis or the presence of a lesion. Being able to glide low but not high often means a lesion is preventing the fold(s) from elongating and thinning enough to vibrate in the upper register. Dynamics also play into evaluating your problem. If singing softly is impossible, then nodules, a polyp, swelling, or muscle tension dysphonia may be at fault. (See 10.15 Muscle Tension Dysphonia.)

In addition to these exercises, common requests are for the patient to talk and sing problematic passages. If you have a specific problem or struggle with an area of your range or *passaggio*, request that the study include an evaluation of that problem so that you and the clinician can observe what is happening. This allows for immediate feedback regarding what is occurring. Together, you can discuss and observe what the clinician is seeing as she assesses motion, vibration, or pathologies; the stability of the laryngeal position; tongue base retraction; and narrowing of the resonating space in the larynx. A really thorough exam could include both oral and nasal endoscopy.

9

A Partnership in Performance

▶ AFTER COMPLETING THIS chapter, you will be ready to view video clips 1 through 5 on the companion website: www.oup.com/us/ownersmanualtothevoice.

9.1 DIAGNOSE WITH THE DOCTOR—DON'T BE LEFT OUT!

Don't be afraid to ask the physicians and clinicians anything. Their job is to help you get better, but they are also there to educate and help you understand vocal health. You must be your own best advocate! You'll only benefit from asking questions, observing your vocal folds with them, and knowing what they're looking at.

9.2 HOW VOICE SPECIALISTS SEE YOUR INSTRUMENT

Figures 9.2a and 9.2b depict pictures of a healthy larynx obtained with an oral endoscope. To capture these images, the endoscope was inserted into the mouth to peer over and behind the tongue, allowing a **sublingual** (below the tongue) and supraglottal (above the glottis) view down into the larynx from above. Remember, laryngeal imaging is magnified. The vocal folds average 15 to 18 mm (only slightly longer than the white half-moons on your fingernails) and are difficult to observe without magnification. The clinician faces the patient to insert the scope. The image that the scope picks up is viewed as though you're facing that person; thus, the left vocal fold in the picture is actually the right vocal fold and vice versa.

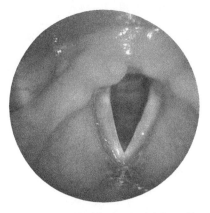

FIGURE 9.2a Healthy Larynx (abducted)
Halogen lighting, abducted normal vocal folds. Person is breathing.

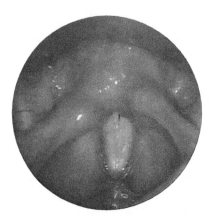

FIGURE 9.2b Healthy Larynx (adducted)
Another normal pair of vocal folds, this time adducted and phonating. Nice closure and well-retracted false folds during phonation. Slight mutational chink suggests that this patient is a female.

Note: The folds appear whitish rather than pink, because the white ligament is what shows through the transparent cover layers, and the ligament doesn't contain any blood-carrying capillaries. The capillaries that exist in the superficial lamina propria above the ligament are extremely tiny and thin. Although these blood vessels are more prominent in some people, they are often only visible when the folds are irritated. An irritation to the vocal folds will cause them to fill up with more blood and give the folds a more **vascular** appearance.

Note: Some clinicians turn the image upside down when showing the patient, so that right is right and left is left. This can get confusing! If it is unclear, you can make a "V" with your fingers and point the "V" into your own neck.

Let's map what we see. The right and left diagonal lines that form a whitish "V" in the center of the photos are the vocal folds. There are only two vocal folds. In Figure 9.2a they are abducted, allowing air to pass in and out of the trachea below.

Note: Can you make out a couple cartilage rings of the trachea below the vocal folds? If not, see Figures 10.6a, 10.7b, and 10.12.

In Figure 9.2b the folds are adducted and phonating. Because the anterior commissure is directly behind and just below the thyroid notch, the bottom of the photo is toward the front of the neck. Sometimes, clinicians will point to the top of the picture and call it the back of the neck, simply to orient the patient. Remember, however, the larynx only takes up a few inches in the front of the neck, so the top of the picture would more accurately be described as being toward the middle of the neck. The faint horizontal line behind the larynx at the very top of the photos is where the larynx meets the pharyngeal wall. If you were to separate the tissue on either side of the line, you'd see the opening to the esophagus (**upper esophageal sphincter [UES]**).

Because we're looking down on top of the folds, we're not able to see their depth. From this perspective we also cannot see the laryngeal ventricle between the true whitish folds and the pink false folds running parallel just above and to the sides.

The clinician begins by listening. She should let you talk about your problem, and she will ask you questions. Often you will be asked to vocalize to allow assessment of your vocal quality. Areas that are observed include your breathing technique, the volume and pitch of your speaking voice, and, if you come prepared to sing, your singing as well. Be sure to bring some music or at the very least have some songs in mind to demonstrate problem areas. Once a brief qualitative evaluation is completed, a visual assessment begins using either a nasendoscope or oral endoscope to magnify and brightly illuminate the folds with the halogen light. When the image of your vocal folds appears on the monitor, the clinician makes a number of observations. The folds are evaluated for superficial hydration, making sure the mucus is thin and plentiful. The clinician can tell if you're not hydrated when the mucus is more sticky than wet and if it beads or strings. (See Figures 10.7a and 10.14.) She then evaluates the colors and symmetry of the vocal folds, as well as the structures surrounding the larynx. Are the folds whitish and surrounded by light pink tissue? Are they the same length and width? Or are they swollen, gray, or threaded with enlarged capillaries and bordered with abnormally red surrounding tissues? She checks that the arytenoid cartilages are symmetrical and that the **interarytenoid space**, as well as the area between the back of the larynx and the esophagus, doesn't display visible evidence of reflux (e.g., thick, swollen, and wrinkled interarytenoid tissue and swollen tissue behind the larynx known as posterior cricoid edema).

Note: The true vocal folds are not a pure, bleached white, which is why we use "whitish" to describe them.

The majority of the exam and final part of the evaluation are spent closely observing the functioning characteristics of the vocal folds under the strobe light. This part of the exam is called videostroboscopy.

The arytenoids should simultaneously swivel to adduct the folds, bringing them together without overlapping. As the two folds begin to phonate, the vibratory pattern is evaluated. The lip-like edges of the folds should roll closed from bottom to top while the edges seal like a Ziploc® from front to back in smooth wave-like motions. (See Video 5.) The clinician makes sure that the false folds' movements are passive during sustained phonation (e.g., held vowel sounds). She knows that if they try to approximate during sustained phonation, they will place unnecessary tension on the true folds and impede their free, healthy, vibratory motion.

Note: We have observed that the false folds are actually retracted out of the way during most healthy singing, allowing the true folds their maximum freedom of vibration. (See Figure 9.2b.) We've also observed, however, that to produce a healthy twang (think Alison Kraus or Kristin Chenoweth) and some high-intensity singing, the **aryepiglottic sphincter** contracts, narrowing the laryngeal vestibule, and the false folds are *passively* brought closer together as room becomes limited. An experienced clinician will be able to *hear* whether false fold medialization is passive or due to muscular contraction, because false fold contraction during phonation causes the voice to sound pressed or strained. (See Figure 10.15.)

The clinician evaluates the closed and open phases of each vibratory cycle. She looks for vocal fold flexibility during the open phase and the vocal folds' ability to make contact and close during the closed phase. She uses the strobe's zero phase option to capture the folds just as they begin to enter their closed phase, so that she can catch a clear view of the folds' lower portion.

Note: The term "phase" is used in clinics in two different ways: to refer to the vocal folds' phases or to refer to the strobe light's phases. This can be confusing! Earlier we used the term "phase" to refer to the times in which your vocal folds are open or closed during each vibratory cycle. And later in Chapter 10 you will be introduced to pathologies that cause the folds to vibrate "**out of phase**" with each other. However, here we use "phase" to refer to the setting options of the strobe's flash.

The appearance of a moist, periodic cover wave means the superficial lamina propria is providing ample cushioning during phonation and thus reveals whether or not the patient practices good long-term hydration habits. When the cover layers are well hydrated, the folds are able to adhere together to seal out excess air during phonation, as well as stretch like elastic for high notes.

Note: Although it is a big indicator, a lack of cover wave does not *always* mean that the folds are dehydrated or unhealthy. The presence of a cover wave tends to appear less in hooty voices, such as those heard in boy choirs, in which the epithelium is pulled taut for an acoustical effect.

The medial or **free edges** of the vocal folds are the most important ingredient for clean sound production. The contact between the two opposing edges is assessed for symmetry, degree of closure, and vibratory characteristics. Are there any gaps in the closure or an abnormally large **mutational chink** through which air is leaking? (In breathy phonation, the vocal folds rarely make contact and there may be an area where the folds aren't coming together.) Are there any lesions or abnormalities along the medial edges that interrupt the folds' closure?

For the clinician to accurately notate and address specific observations along the vocal folds, a numbering system is often used. The vocal folds are sectioned into thirds and numbered 1 through 9 from front to back. (See Figure 9.2c.) Numbers 1 through 3 mark the anterior one-third portion of the folds nearest the anterior commissure, 4 through 6 mark the middle third, and 7 through 9 make up the posterior third where the folds thin and cover an extension of the arytenoid cartilage called the **vocal process**.

The junction of the anterior one third and the posterior two thirds of the vocal folds is of particular concern and is closely evaluated by the clinician. This area between 3 and 4, also known as the midmembranous portion of the folds, is examined carefully because this is where the vocal folds take the brunt of each vibration. Because of the stress to this area, the midmembranous portion is a pathology hotspot where most

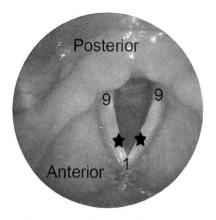

FIGURE 9.2C Reference Points on the Vocal Folds
The numbers 1 through 9 are used to refer to the areas along each fold. In this picture, the number 9s are enlarged for visibility and actually cover the entire vocal processes 7 through 9. The stars mark 3 to 4 or the point of maximum glottal contact.

vocal fold lesions form. Premature contact at this junction often implies faulty singing technique, as well as the imminent formation of nodules. We will refer to this susceptible area as the "**point of maximum glottal contact**" or **PMGC** throughout the book.[1]

Note: Physicians are quick to explain the midmembranous portion of the folds as the "point of the greatest vocal excursion." So, what do they mean? Visualize the folds for a minute. Because the posterior third of the folds is only epithelium and basement membrane over cartilage (the arytenoid's vocal process), this portion of the folds is stiff and doesn't vibrate. Only the front two thirds of the vocal folds actually vibrate. This means the halfway mark of the vibrating portion is actually between 3 and 4! Once you understand that the area between 3 and 4 is really the middle of the *vibrating* fold, you know it is the point farthest away from the fixed ends of the fold and is therefore the freest-moving portion of the fold. Because it is the freest, it is propelled in and out of the glottis the farthest and gets "banged around" the most during vibration. As the midmembranous portions of the folds crash together, they become the most susceptible points along the folds to getting bruised or developing another type of impact lesion.

---

[1] Although "the midmembranous portion of the folds" is commonly used by medical specialists in the field, we prefer the simplified and descriptive, though nontraditional, "PMGC."

Note: We've noticed that nodules and other lesions in classical singers tend to develop around 4 or even between 4 and 5, rather than the typical area of 3 to 4. Perhaps because a classical singer spends so much time sustaining phonation in the upper register of a three-octave range, the folds remain in an elongated state and the location of the PMGC moves closer to 4 and 5.

9.3 SEMANTICS

Much of our voice studio terminology is figurative, based on imagery and subjective opinion rather than scientific measurement. In the studio, we have the luxury of sharing a common slang vocabulary with each other to describe what we feel and hear. Though not scientific, this vocabulary is virtually universal among classically trained singers and instructors. To avoid confusion, we need to share a vocabulary with our laryngologist as well. These next four sections are geared toward clarifying vocabulary so that we can communicate intelligently and efficiently together. Let's begin with a few words commonly misstated or misunderstood by singers when talking with the laryngologist.

Analgesic versus anesthetic

An anesthetic is an over-the-counter or prescription drug that numbs or reduces sensation. Cepacol® throat lozenges reduce not only throat soreness but also throat sensation because they contain a mild anesthetic. An **analgesic** is an over-the-counter or prescription drug that reduces pain but still allows sensation to be felt, such as Tylenol®.

Aspirate versus aspirate onset

The word "aspirate" has two different pronunciations and meanings, depending on whether it's used as a verb or as an adjective. To **aspirate** (a-spur-ATE) means to inhale something other than air into the lungs. You may also hear it used when food or liquid enters the airway. Patients who have difficulty swallowing may be described as aspirating when liquid or food pools in their larynx and causes them to produce an occasional gargled sound or a choke while breathing or talking. A person can also aspirate if the airway is unprotected (e.g., talking with a mouthful of food or eating with a vocal fold paralysis). To aspirate is to have something "go down the wrong pipe."

To aspirate (a-spur-ATE) can also mean to begin a sound with air escaping audibly between approximated folds. We "a-spur-ATE" the consonant "h". However, aspirate is pronounced "a-spur-IT" when used as an adjective describing this breathy beginning to a sound. When breath escapes before a tone, as in "he," the onset of that tone is described as an "a-spur-IT" onset.

Breathy versus hoarse

These descriptions for voice quality are often used interchangeably by the average Joe, but they are not synonymous. Breathiness occurs when the vocal folds don't come together sufficiently during phonation, allowing air to escape. General muscle weakness or laziness at the lung or vocal fold level may not sufficiently power phonation, and a soft, breathy voice will be the result. A large glottal gap, mutational chink, or pathology such as a **paralysis** or lesion can also be culprits causing breathiness. A breathy tone, however, can still be clean and clear in quality à la Marilyn Monroe, Sade, and Enya. A hoarse voice is a combination of breathiness and roughness. Hoarseness is caused by vocal fold stiffness, whether from swelling or a paralysis, combined with muscle tension as the person strains to compensate. The clarity of the tone is compromised and has a raspy quality to it à la Demi Moore and Bill Clinton.

Note: It is important to note that when a true physical muscular weakness such as muscular dystrophy (MS) causes a soft, breathy voice, the voice is called **asthenic**.

Elastic rebound versus elastic recoil

These terms are not interchangeable. Elastic rebound is a theory used to explain how two surfaces in the earth can grind together and result in an earthquake. Elastic rebound has nothing to do with the voice. Elastic recoil generally describes the flexible characteristics of soft tissue and muscle. Once any muscle releases its contraction, it wants to spring back to its resting position. A good example are the rib muscles that want to torque back down after expanding out and up for inhalation.

Hypertension versus hyperfunction

Hypo- and hypertension refer to blood pressure, not to the voice. Hypo- and hyperfunction are terms used to describe voice production. Allowing the voice to fall into glottal fry at the ends of sentences is a result of allowing laryngeal and voice musculature to hypofunction (underenergize). As we age, our muscles weaken and our voices become more hypofunctioning as well. A loud whisper causes laryngeal and voice musculature to hyperfunction (overenergize), as does cheerleading and yelling for the dog to come in.

Intensity versus loudness

Intensity is the objective measurement of sound strength in decibels (dB), whereas loudness is the subjective human perception of sound strength.

Fundamental frequency versus pitch

When used in regard to the voice, the term "fundamental frequency" is basically the *number* of times the vocal folds vibrate per second. It is the *objective measurement* of the vocal folds', or any sound-generating device's, periodic vibrating rate. The pitch, on the other hand, is what the human ear perceives. The pitch is the *perceptual aspect* of the fundamental frequency. In other words, if you hear the pitch "A4," something is producing a fundamental frequency of (vibrating at) 440 cycles per second (cps).[2]

Note: Singers sometimes refer casually to the fundamental frequency as "the fundamental."

Note: "A440" is typically the pitch to which pianos are tuned.

Jitter

Singers might use the word "jitter" to describe shakiness or uneven vibrato in the voice. However, using "jitter" to subjectively describe a quality heard in a voice could confuse ENT clinicians. ENT clinicians use the term to refer to minute, but measurable, variations that randomly occur within the wave of each vocal fold vibration. Clinicians use special equipment to measure the amounts of jitter in a person's voice while that person tries to produce a steady tone. All voices have some degree of jitter. Slight variations in vibrations normally occur that alter the frequency or pitch very briefly. It is not clear whether normal degrees of jitter can be perceived by our ears. As jitter increases, however, the interference to frequency increases and begins to detract from the sound quality, producing noise. Noise is perceptible to the human ear and is commonly described as roughness.

Shimmer

You might use "**shimmer**" to describe a positive perceptual attribute of the singing voice (e.g., "Her voice has a beautiful shimmer to it"). However, as with jitter, using "shimmer" to describe a perceived voice quality may confuse ENT clinicians who recognize shimmer as a measurable variation in the vocal folds' **lateral excursion** from the midline with each vibration. Simply put, shimmer is a rapid fluctuation in the loudness of a voice. All naturally produced voices include some degree of shimmer, and although normal degrees

---

[2] We're assuming that middle C—the fourth C from the bottom of the piano keyboard—is C4, so A4 would be the A above middle C.

of fluctuation can be objectively measured, it is not clear whether they are audible. As shimmer increases, however, it produces noise that is perceptible to the human ear and commonly described as roughness.

Vestibule versus ventricle

The false folds can also be correctly referred to as vestibular folds or ventricular folds. However, a **vestibule** and a ventricle are different things. A ventricle is any small recess or hollow space, whereas a vestibule is a hollow space forming the entry to a canal. You may conclude that all vestibules are ventricles, but not all ventricles are vestibules. With regard to the larynx, the ventricle refers to the cavity just below and lateral to the false folds, above the true folds. This space must be unobstructed to allow the true vocal folds to vibrate freely. On the other hand, the larynx's vestibule is the opening of the larynx and the hollow area just above the false folds within the aryepiglottic sphincter. Therefore, by referring to the false folds as ventricular folds or vestibular folds, you are simply choosing between two ways of depicting their same location in the larynx.

Mucous membrane vs. mucosa vs. mucus vs. mucous

Mucous membrane and mucosa are synonymous nouns referring to the type of tissue that secretes clear lubricating fluid called mucus. Mucosa lines the mouth, nose, pharynx, larynx, true and false folds, trachea, lungs, urogenital tract, reproductive organs, esophagus, and gastrointestinal (GI) tract. Mucous (ending in "o-u-s") is the adjective spelling, as in mucous membrane.

Mucus vs. saliva

All saliva is mucus, but not all mucus is saliva. All salivary glands are along the digestive tract. There are major groupings of salivary glands in the mouth and smaller, minor salivary glands on the roof of the mouth and throughout the throat and larynx. Saliva contains digestive enzymes, and its consistency depends on the enzymes it needs to break the food down that you take into your mouth. Mucus is in the nose and is influenced by the environment (the dry heat inside and cold air outside in the winter, for example). You can alter the consistency of your mucus based on your day-to-day water intake. Saliva is not as influenced by day-to-day water intake as it is by medications and diet. Medications that dry out the mouth badly will not affect the mucus in the nose to the same extreme, for example.

Vocal fold vs. vocal ligament, thyroarytenoid muscles, and vocalis

People incorrectly use these three terms interchangeably, when in fact the latter three refer to specific parts within the vocal folds. Each true vocal fold contains a vocal ligament in its middle or transition layer. Each true fold also contains a muscular layer. Muscles are named for their number (biceps, triceps), shape (trapezius), size (gluteus maximus), location (intercostals, meaning "between ribs"), or, in the case of the thyroarytenoid muscles, attachments. When you hear clinicians use the term "thyroarytenoid muscles," they are referring to a group of muscles that originate at the thyroid cartilage and insert at the arytenoids within each vocal fold. The thyroarytenoid muscles can be broken down into two distinct bands of muscles: the medial thyroarytenoid muscle (a.k.a. the vocalis muscle) and the lateral thyroarytenoid muscle (a.k.a. the thyromuscularis).

> Note: The thyromuscularis is not as nice and neat as the band of muscle pictured in Figure 2.2i and its actions are not certain. Many believe it contracts and, to a lesser degree than the vocalis, contributes to shortening the folds and relaxing the vocal fold cover. However, some of its fibers contribute to form nearly a complete ring around the glottis suggesting that it may also contribute to the sphincter function of the laryngeal vestibule.

Attack vs. onset

Singers often use the term "attack" to mean vocal onset, as in "glottal attack." However, this use of the term may confuse clinicians, who sometimes use "glottal attack" to refer to any harsh slamming of the folds, whether verbal or a hard cough. The term "onset" is used by clinicians to refer to the initiation of phonation and is a better choice when speaking with them.

TMJ vs. TMJ dysfunction

Laypeople often use the acronym **TMJ** to refer to a chronic problem with pain or limited movement in the jaw; however, this is technically incorrect. TMJ refers to the **temporomandibular joint** only. To convey that you have a joint condition, it's correct to say, "I have TMJ dysfunction (or a TMJ disorder)" or "I have TMD." **Temporomandibular joint dysfunction** (**TMD**) is often due to disc displacement, a form of arthritis in the jaw joint, or a tear in the **meniscus** of the jaw joint (similar to what can happen in the knee joint).

Adam's apple versus thyroid notch

Many people use these terms interchangeably to refer to the prominence at the front of the neck. The Adam's apple, however, refers to the lateral (left to right) angle of the thyroid cartilage prominence, whereas "thyroid notch" denotes the dip in the middle of the cartilage. The notch becomes deeper and the prominence more pronounced in a male's thyroid cartilage during puberty. This change in the cartilage plays a part in the instability of the pubescent male voice.

Laryngitis versus hoarseness

Some people may incorrectly use the term "laryngitis" to refer to any hoarseness or complete loss of voice. The "-itis" suffix of the word dictates inflammation. Laryngitis is any laryngeal inflammation, whether brought on by a misuse, overuse, irritation, or infection. Although hoarseness and loss of voice are the common symptoms of laryngitis, they can also be symptoms of several other laryngeal pathologies and disorders. For instance, a vocal fold paresis or bowing that results in hoarseness should not be referred to as laryngitis.

9.4 SYNONYMS: A ROSETTA STONE FOR VOICE AND MEDICAL PROFESSIONALS

To follow is a list of words that can be used interchangeably. Where applicable, terms are distinguished by their use. Boldface terms are often **used by medical professionals**. Italicized terms are *common to singers*. Those underlined are layperson or slang terms.

1. **agent**/ingredient
2. **aspirate onset**/*breathy attack*/soft onset/blown onset
3. **basement membrane/basal lamina**
4. **bowed vocal folds/myasthenia laryngis**/muscular atrophy
5. *costal breath/thoracic breath/chest breath*/"breathing with your chest"
6. **cranial/rostral/**toward the head
7. **cricothyroid membrane/conus elasticus/lateral cricothyroid ligaments**
8. *thoracic-abdominal breath/combination breath/balanced breath/abdominal breath/*low breath*/belly breath/"breathing with your diaphragm"*
9. **diplophonia**/biphonia/two tone
10. **dysphonia/**hoarseness
11. *easy onset/simultaneous onset*/gentle onset/balanced onset
12. **edema/fluid retention/**swelling/bloating
13. **endotracheal tube (ETT)/intubation tube/**breathing tube
14. **epidermis/**skin
15. **epithelium/epithelial layer/epithelial lining**
16. *esophagus/***alimentary canal/**food chute
17. **frequency range/***vocal range/*pitch range
18. **functional dysphonia/conversion dysphonia/psychogenic dysphonia/**hysterical dysphonia (or aphonia)

19. *glottal fry*/*vocal fry*/<u>creak voice</u>/pulse register
20. **glottal gap/glottic gap/glottal chink/glottic chink**
21. **glottal onset**/hard onset/*glottal attack*/*coup de glotte*/glottal stop/stroke of the glottis
22. **glottis**/rima glottidis
23. **hemorrhage**/*<u>bruise</u>*/burst blood vessel
24. **hertz**/Hz/<u>cycles per second</u>/cps
25. **intensity range**/dynamic range
26. **interarytenoideus/arytenoideus**
27. **laryngeal prominence**/<u>Adam's apple</u>
28. **laryngeal saccule**/appendix of the laryngeal ventricle/laryngeal pouch/Hilton's pouch
29. **laryngeal vestibule/epilarynx**/laryngeal tube/supraglottis
30. **laryngologist/phonosurgeon**/<u>voice doctor</u>/*ENT*
31. *laryngopharynx*/**hypopharynx**
32. **larynx**/*vocal mechanism*/<u>voice box</u>/vocal apparatus
33. *lutta vocale*/breath opposition/vocal struggle
34. **microlaryngeal surgery/laryngeal microsurgery**
35. **mucosa/mucous membrane/mucosal lining**
36. **muscle tension dysphonia/MTD/hyperkinetic vocal function**
37. **nasendoscopy**/transnasal fiberoptic laryngoscopy
38. *oral cavity*/**buccal cavity**/albicans/<u>mouth</u>
39. **otolaryngologist**/<u>ear, nose, and throat doctor</u>/ENT
40. **otolaryngology**/<u>ear, nose, and throat</u>/otorhinolaryngology
41. **paradoxical vocal fold movement/PVFM/vocal cord dysfunction/VCD**
42. **pharmacopoeia**/*<u>list of drugs</u>*/collection of drugs
43. **pharyngeal ostium (opening) of the ear/orifice of auditory tube**/eustachian tube entrance
44. **pharynx**/*<u>throat</u>*
45. **phonotrauma/vocal trauma**
46. **polypoid corditis/polypoid degeneration/Reinke's edema**/*<u>smoker's voice</u>*
47. **presbylarynx/presbylaringes**
48. **puberphonia**/*mutational falsetto*/incomplete mutation/adolescent transitional dysphonia
49. **rectus**/<u>straight</u>
50. **resonating cavities**/*vocal tract*/resonating tract
51. **serous mucus**/thin mucus
52. *soft palate*/muscular palate
53. **sternum**/<u>breastbone</u>
54. *subglottal*/**subglottic**
55. *thorax*/*<u>torso</u>*/chest

56. **thyroarytenoid muscles**/*body of the vocal folds*
57. **thyromuscularis**/**lateral thyroarytenoid**/pars muscularis/muscularis
58. **trachea**/<u>windpipe</u>
59. *uvula*/palatine uvula
60. **Valsalva maneuver**/*thoracic fixation*/abdominal fixation
61. **varix**/<u>varicose vein</u>/blood vessel prominence
62. **ventricle/ventricular sinus/ventricular vestibule/laryngeal sinus/Morgagni's ventricle/sinus of Morgagni**
63. **vestibular folds/ventricular folds**/*false folds*/false vocal cords
64. **vibratory cycle/period/cycle**
65. **video laryngeal stroboscopy/VLS/videostroboscopy**/strobolaryngoscopy
66. **viscous mucus**/*phlegm*/thick mucus
67. **vocal folds/true vocal folds**/*vocal cords/cords*
68. *vocal ligament*/**thyroarytenoid ligament**
69. **vocal performer**/*singer*/vocalist
70. **vocalis**/*vocalis muscle*/pars vocalis/thyrovocalis/medial thyroarytenoid
71. *voice therapy*/**vocal rehabilitation**
72. *voice clinic*/<u>*ENT clinic*</u>/speech and hearing clinic
73. **zero phase/phase lock**

9.5 MISNOMERS

The following terms are terms accepted and adopted through habit but don't necessarily reflect the definition of the word accurately.

Pachyderma/pachydermia

The term interarytenoid *pachyderma* or *pachydermia* is used by medical specialists to refer to laryngeal tissue that has been repeatedly irritated by refluxed stomach acid, inhaler use, smoking, or postnasal drainage. Evidence of pachyderma is apparent due to its whitish gray color and wrinkled, tethered thickness left by repeated or frequent irritation. Pachyderma breaks down in Greek to literally mean "thick skin" (*pachy* means "thick"; *dermatos* means "skin"). However, because the tissue that lines the larynx (including the interarytenoid area) is not skin but actually mucous membrane, using the term pachyderma when referring to laryngeal tissue is technically incorrect. If you want to impress, attach the Latin suffix "-menia," meaning membrane, and say pachymenia instead!

Note: A pachyderm is any thick-skinned mammal such as an elephant, hippopotamus, or rhinoceros.

Bilateral nodules

To say "bilateral nodules" (meaning there is one on each of the two vocal folds) is redundant. Nodules are always parallel and always in pairs. Some physicians, however, use the word "nodule" to generically refer to any bump-like lesion (such as a polyp or cyst) until they are sure of the type of lesion it is. Such physicians may therefore refer to bilateral lesions as bilateral "nodules" until a thorough evaluation determines exactly what type lesions they are. Actual nodules are bilateral and symmetric. If the lesions do not look the same in size and shape, they are most likely not nodules. (See Figures 10.5a and 10.5b.)

Sympathetic "resonance"

There is no such thing as a sympathetic resonator. Something either is a resonator or is not. Some singers mistakenly use the words "sympathetic resonance" when referring to sensations felt in areas other than those actually resonating (e.g., "chest resonance"). However, resonance occurs only when sound waves directly fill an acoustic space. Our sounds can only resonate in the pharynx, mouth, nose, and sinuses. Anything we feel outside of these resonators during phonation is sympathetic *vibration*. We are all built and wired up a bit differently, and what we feel will differ slightly. Transmissions of the voice's vibration can be conducted through the body's tissues and felt in the bones, Eustachian tubes, ears, chest, and even fingertips for some! Even using the term "mask resonance," common among singers, is tricky. A lot of the sensation felt in the mask during resonant singing and speaking is really sympathetic vibration. Sensations felt behind the eyes while singing are sympathetic vibrations, for instance. Sensations felt in the nose and sinuses are as well if the soft palate is raised while singing, as this prevents sound waves from entering the nose and sinuses. Perhaps it would be better to say "mask vibrations" rather than "mask resonance."

Reinke's "space"

To call the vocal fold's superficial lamina propria layer by its other name, "Reinke's space," is less accurate. The layer isn't actually an empty space. Lying below the epithelium's basement membrane and above the vocal ligament, this layer contains loosely bound tissue fibers, some tiny capillaries, and gel-like fluid. Even when dehydrated, and the water component of the gel becomes depleted, the layer never completely empties and becomes space. The authors, therefore, prefer the term "superficial lamina propria." (See 3.6 Vocal Maintenance.)

"Edges" of the true vocal folds

Although very commonly used in voice literature among medical professionals, the term "edge" is somewhat of a misnomer when referring to the vocal fold's free inner margin. The vocal folds' "edges" are actually rounded somewhat like lips and, when vibrating, present an upper and lower portion of lip. We think that saying "medial lips," "the free portions of the folds," or "the **free margins** of the vocal folds" might be a more accurate way of referring to the edges; however, we have still elected to use the term "edge" throughout this book. We feel the term "edge" better describes what you see in two-dimensional laryngoscopic still photos of the vocal folds and is often easier to picture than "lips" or "margins" when describing details on the folds.

Voice therapist/voice pathologist/speech therapist/speech pathologist

While these titles are often used interchangeably for all who have at least a master's degree in speech-language pathology, speech-language pathologist (SLP) is the only official title recognized by the American Speech-Language-Hearing Association (ASHA) for these clinicians. SLPs are professionals who are educated to assist in speech-language development and disorders and can also help with swallowing and voice disorders. SLPs who use their degree to work in schools with children's speech may prefer a shorter, simpler title such as speech therapists. SLPs who use their certification to focus on voice in particular may even have a vocal performance degree and refer to themselves by a title more indicative of their skills, such as "clinical voice pathologists."

Throat = vocal folds

Although we may colloquially use "throat" to refer to the back of the mouth down to the larynx and esophagus, many singers wrongly use the term "throat" to refer specifically to the vocal folds. The throat is actually a long continuous space called the pharynx that extends up from the back of the mouth, as well as down! The pharynx, or throat, begins behind the nose (nasopharynx) and runs down behind the soft palate, down the back of the mouth (oropharynx), and continues down further behind and below the tongue, until it reaches the portion of the throat in and just behind the larynx (laryngopharynx). The pharynx ends at the vocal folds and the top of the esophagus. The vocal folds are located at the bottom of the laryngopharynx in the laryngeal vestibule, just anterior to the esophageal opening. (See Figures 2.2g, 2.2h, 2.2j, and 5.10.)

9.6 TERMS TO AVOID

Although the following terms are universally understood and often even used by physicians when communicating with a novice patient, there are better choices to make you sound more informed.

ENT

Otolaryngologists and laryngologists generally do not like to be called "ENTs." The acronym is more appropriately used to refer to the ENT (ear, nose, and throat) clinic and not the person.

Node or nodes

There is no such thing as a "node" when referring to vocal fold nodules. To say "nodes" is grammatically incorrect. "Nodules" is the correct term and will always be plural because nodules occur in pairs.

Vocal cords

To say "vocal *cords*" is to misrepresent our multilayered instrument. When observed from above, our instrument may appear to look like simple whitish strips of cord, but when viewed from the side, they have depth. Each vocal fold has a flat upper (superior) surface and a curved sloping medial lip that tapers into its lower (inferior) surface, making its shape more like an exaggerated airplane wing, not a cord. Each fold is also unlike a cord in that each contains a variety of layers and isn't a white strip like it appears to be. When air passes between the two adducted folds for phonation, the looser outside layer rhythmically slips and slides over the inner layers while appearing on the outside like a wave in water with each vibration. This complex pattern is very different than air passing between two strings or cords, which would resemble more of a reed instrument. (Picture blowing on a blade of grass held between your thumbs.) Our instrument is thus more accurately referred to as vocal folds.

> Note: When referring to laryngeal anatomy, cord is spelled differently than the triadic chord with a "c-h" that is played on a piano or guitar.

Voice box

It is better to say larynx.

"LARE-niks"

The word "larynx" is very commonly mispronounced by not only laypeople but also doctors and nurses! The correct pronunciation of larynx is "LARE-ringks." Notice that the "y" comes before the "n." Think "larynx and pharynx rhyme with sphinx," and you won't go wrong.

10

Common Pathologies and Disorders in Singers and

Possible Treatments

VOICE PATHOLOGIES AND disorders fall under many categories and combinations of categories. They may be something that you are born with and may or may not be genetic (**congenital**), or they may not be genetic at all and develop later in life (**acquired**). They may be characterized as stemming from **vocal hyperfunction** or **vocal hypofunction**, meaning that too much or too little physical effort is being used when phonating, respectively. They may be further described as occurring suddenly (acute), such as a lesion erupting from a one-time occurrence of the vocal mechanism being employed in an inefficient and harsh manner (vocal misuse), like one loud yell or hard cough. Alternatively, they may develop, persist, and recur over time (chronic), perhaps stemming from bad vocal habits (vocal abuse), like speaking too loudly too often or habitually clearing the throat.

> Note: Some clinicians prefer to use the more general and emotionally neutral term "**phonotrauma**" or "phonotraumatic behavior" when talking to a patient about his tendency to talk too loudly, for instance. We choose to use the common though agreeably harsher-sounding terms vocal "misuse" and "abuse" to clearly differentiate between types of phonotraumas in this book.

It is important to note a few other descriptive terms voice medical professionals use when referring to the nature of ailments. Pathologies and disorders relating to the organs of the body are *organic*, those relating to the moving and functioning of the body are *functional*, those relating to personal behaviors are *behavioral*, and those relating to the nervous system are *neurological*. While these terms are commonly used among voice specialists and in voice literature, some of their meanings and applications are blurred. Because the larynx is an organ, anything affecting it would, by definition, be organic. However, many clinicians use "organic" to refer to disorders where the cause is not due to anything the patient did wrong or had control over (e.g., a congenital disorder, vocal folds bowing with old age, or a vocal fold paralysis from a virus). Many use the term "functional" to refer to disorders that are more psychological in origin, whether conscious or subconscious, and have no identifiable neurological or pathological cause (e.g., a singer who has a recital coming up and suddenly "loses her voice" would be considered to have functional aphonia). Additionally, "nonorganic" is a term sometimes used to describe something caused by a direct vocal trauma (e.g., **intubation** or one hard cough). "Behavioral" is used to describe a lesion that developed from a habit or something the patient did one time (e.g., a polyp from a big yell or nodules from talking too loudly all the time) and is sometimes used interchangeably with "acquired." Another term, "nonacquired," may describe something congenital or viral. "Psychiatric" implies that the disorder is directly related to an underlying mental health reason (e.g., muscle tension dysphonia, psychogenic voice loss, or paradoxical vocal fold movement [PVFM] due to stress, repressed memories, or a history of abuse or depression). Classifications are problematic: a particular issue may fit many classifications, a classification may have more than one meaning, and there are many areas of overlap. To give one example as to why these classifications can be cumbersome to use: **Polypoid corditis**, as you will learn more about in this chapter, can develop from inhaling too much of an irritant. If the patient is an auto mechanic and the irritant is exhaust exposure, the pathology is considered organic. But if a problem is induced by smoking, the pathology is considered to be caused by abusive behavior and can be considered behavioral. Because the applications of these classifying terms are inconsistent in the literature and because pathologies and disorders can fall under more than one of these classes, we have not relied on them to describe the ailments in this chapter. We mention them only to make the reader aware of their meanings and common use in the clinic. The pathologies and disorders described in this chapter are broken down by the following questions:

a. What is it? (Pathology or disorder definition)
b. How can you tell if you have it? (Symptoms)
   Visually (visible distinctions)
   Audibly (audible characteristics)
   Production variations (changes in vocal effort and sensations)
c. How do you get it? (Causes/**etiology**)
d. Who's susceptible? (What puts someone at risk?)
e. How is it fixed? (Treatment options)

The information presented here is for self-edification and not a substitute for professional care. It is difficult to self-diagnose the disorder or pathology you have based on the symptoms alone! Visualization and assessment by a qualified team that specializes in voice is always best.

10.1 LARYNGEAL EDEMA AND ERYTHEMA

What is it?

- *Edema* is the medical term for swelling. It denotes protein-bound water buildup that has formed as a protective cushion under an injured or inflamed lining. Edema is the earliest evidence of excessive irritation to or inflammation of the vocal fold.

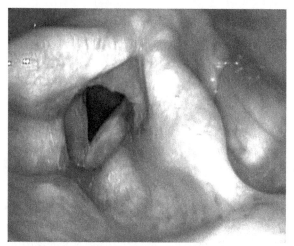

FIGURE 10.1a Laryngeal Edema and Erythema (abducted)
Halogen lighting. Bilateral vocal fold edema and erythema (right fold is especially erythematic), nondistinct arytenoids due to swelling. Obvious interarytenoid pachyderma.

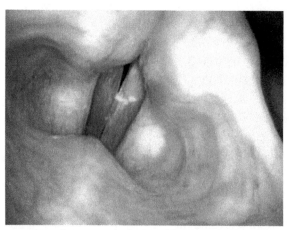

FIGURE 10.1b Laryngeal Edema and Erythema (adducted)
Xenon lighting. Significant posterior gap 6 to 9 and slight anterior gap 1 to 2 during phonation due to swelling.

- *Erythema* is the medical term for unusual redness due to some kind of inflammation.
- See Figures 10.1a and 10.1b.

Note: Significant erythema and edema may be classified as laryngitis, depending on the cause.

How can you tell if you have it?

- Audibly: Hoarseness, deep throaty voice, loss of flexibility and range
- Visually: The two conditions can appear together or separately. Edematous laryngeal tissue has a puffy look, and erythematic tissue is abnormally red and inflamed and/or has visible enlarged blood vessels.
- Production variants: Less flexibility, pitch breaks, difficulty with vocal onset (especially in high range), difficulty getting warmed up and staying warmed up

---

Note: An SLP may have you sing a siren sound very quietly from a low pitch to your highest possible pitch or sing "Happy Birthday" as softly and lightly as possible in your higher range to determine the extent of your vocal folds' swelling. Very edematous folds will have much difficulty consistently phonating at a *pianissimo* level in the upper range.

How do you get it?

- An inflammatory reaction triggered any one of the following:
  Infection (cold)
  Premenstrual syndrome (PMS)
  Voice disorder (vocal hyperfunction, stress)
  Behavioral abuse (talking too low or too loudly or smoking)
  Any irritating lesion on the opposite vocal fold
  (If a lesion on one vocal fold's vibrating edge is hard enough, it will irritate the opposite fold during phonation and cause it to redden and swell.)
- If there appears to be swelling between the arytenoids and the esophagus, laryngopharyngeal reflux is the likely culprit.
- If the tissue surrounding the arytenoid joints is erythematic, especially if one is more so than the other, arthritis is the likely culprit.
- Dehydration, sneezing, coughing

Who's susceptible?

- Moms yelling at kids or dog, cheerleaders, animated concertgoers, animated character artists, sports fans, smokers, people who overconsume alcohol regularly, menstruating women the week before their period
- Those who sing when the throat is sore (There are few pain receptors in the larynx, so if you feel pain or even mild discomfort when singing, something is wrong. And remember that throat lozenges can numb the throat, decreasing pharyngeal sensation, and thus prevent you from noticing the discomfort.)
- Untrained professional voice users (teachers, preachers, lawyers, etc.)
- Those with thyroid abnormalities or hormone fluctuation
- Anyone

How is it fixed? (Treatments)

- Hydration, sleep, ibuprofen, voice rest
- If the condition is caused by vocal abuse, it may resolve with voice therapy. An SLP can often identify the abuse and help you stop the abuse with therapy. When in doubt, minimize or abstain from voice use and seek medical attention if the voice does not return within twenty-four hours.
- Vocalizing in a comfortable range and volume, using easy onsets

---

Anecdote: A well-known voice scientist, Katherine Verdolini, was scheduled to have a voice lesson right after work one day. Her teaching schedule and work at the clinic had been particularly busy and vocally taxing, leaving her hoarse and too tired to sing. She scoped herself with the oral endoscope and saw some redness and swelling. When she called to cancel her lesson, however, her teacher didn't answer the phone, so she went to cancel in person. Her teacher urged her to come in despite her vocal complaints, promising just to vocalize her a little. The easy vocalises left Verdolini's voice feeling clear and smooth. Excited, she drove back to clinic after the lesson and scoped herself again. The redness and swelling had visibly improved. Moral: Your voice may tire more quickly from inefficient use than from too much use. How you phonate can affect your voice more than how long you phonate, and good vocalizing can actually help dissipate vocal fold edema and erythema.

Voice Scientist, Katherine Verdolini, PhD, Professor of Communication Science and Disorders in the Department of Otolaryngology, University of Pittsburgh, e-mail message to author, May 25, 2007.

10.2 LARYNGITIS

What is it?

- The general term for inflammation of the larynx. Characterized by hoarseness and "loss of voice" (dysphonia or aphonia) that accompanies inflamed/swollen vocal folds (See Figure 10.2.)

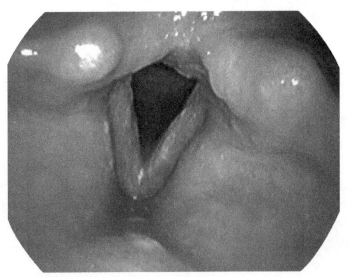

FIGURE 10.2 Laryngitis
General laryngeal edema and erythema. Vocal folds appear inflamed.

- Physicians distinguish between three types:
  Traumatic laryngitis
  Infectious laryngitis
  Noninfectious laryngitis

How can you tell if you have it?
- Audibly: The telltale sign of laryngitis is temporary hoarseness or aphonia. Chronic hoarseness can be a sign of **reflux laryngitis**.
  Gradual onset of hoarseness is a sign of noninfectious laryngitis, caused by allergies, excessive smoking, excessive drinking, or vocal abuse (nodules).
  A sudden inability to phonate well or at all (acute dysphonia or aphonia) is a sign of infectious laryngitis, in which case symptoms should not persist longer than two weeks. If symptoms do persist, see a physician. You may have traumatic laryngitis, in which case a vocal fold pathology stemming from a vocal misuse may be at fault (e.g., polyp, cyst).
- Visually: Laryngeal tissue is edematous, generally erythematic, and may have visible, enlarged blood vessels.
- Production variants: Effortful voice. A raw or tickling sensation and the constant urge to clear the throat accompany dysphonia.

How do you get it?
- Infectious laryngitis can be caused by a viral, bacterial, or fungal infection. Viral infections are usually upper respiratory infections (**URI**s), and bacterial infections are usually lower respiratory infections (**LRI**s).

- Noninfectious laryngitis can be due to rarer conditions such as thyroid disorders but is usually due to reflux. Poor eating habits, weight gain, and late-night eating can lead to repeated acid reflux causing reflux laryngitis.
- Traumatic laryngitis is due to some type of injury, whether self-inflicted, as in an overuse or misuse, or caused by a surgical mishap (**iatrogenic**).

Who's susceptible?
- Anyone

How is it fixed?
- Voice conservation, hydration, and steaming are the treatments for viral laryngitis but only relieve symptoms.
- Antibiotics treat laryngitis brought on by fungal and bacterial infections.

Note: Do not stop taking an antibiotic because you feel better. The dosage given is intended to kill all the bad bacteria, and if you do not finish the prescription, it's possible that enough bad bacteria will remain in your system to make you sick again days or even weeks later!

Note: Do not take an antibiotic before a throat culture. A culture done on antibiotics will not give an accurate reading.

- A nasal saline rinse or a voiceless gargle with saline used during a bacterial infection can reduce the length of time and severity of the infection. Nasal saline is also soothing in that it's effective in flushing the nasal cavity.
- Corticosteroids are prescribed drugs used to mobilize the bound water in the superficial lamina propria and decrease inflammation that accompanies acute inflammatory laryngitis. (See 11.16 Steroids.) Some laryngologists prescribe steroids in low doses. However, for a singer's purposes, a higher dose for a short period of time is more effective. Corticosteroids should be prescribed to singers as a last resort, and ONLY when the singer is committed to performing professionally and inflammation will hinder the performance. Corticosteroids do have some side effects and often make the vocal folds feel heavy. The steroids should not be used more than two or three times a year. If a singer requires more frequent treatment, then the cause of the symptoms should be reexamined.

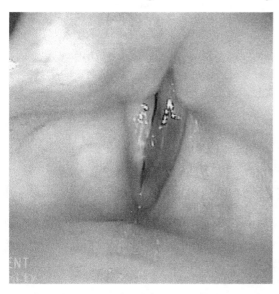

FIGURE 10.3 Vocal Fold
Hemorrhage
Left vocal fold hemorrhage affecting full
length of the fold. Vocal folds adducted and
phonating. Hyaline sessile polyp arising
from 3 to 6 on vibrating edge of left fold
interrupting closure and creating hourglass
appearance.

10.3 VOCAL FOLD HEMORRHAGE

What is it?
- A vocal fold hemorrhage is a ruptured blood vessel bleeding into the vocal fold. (See Figure 10.3.)

How can you tell if you have it?
- Audibly: Blood is heavier than mucus, and a vocal fold with an enlarged or rup-tured capillary will have a greater weight than a normal fold. Two vocal folds of unequal weight will vibrate out of sync with each other, producing a dis-torted hoarse sound. A hemorrhage usually causes dysphonia or aphonia within twenty-four hours of the vocal trauma.
- Visibly: Enlarged or burst blood vessels can appear anywhere on the vocal fold, but often occur at the point of maximum glottal contact (PMGC) (the middle third of the fold).
- Production variants: Loss of flexibility and range. Singers often describe a sensa-tion of a "pop" the moment they feel a fold hemorrhage.

How do you get it?
- Acquired voice disorder due to vocal abuse (excessive voice use), vocal hyperfunc-tion, vocal misuse (e.g., one hard cough, screaming the highest note of a song)

- Dehydration, gastroesophageal reflux disease (GERD), smoking, caffeine, allergies, and excessive alcohol consumption can irritate the folds and leave them in a less than optimal condition to vibrate, predisposing them to hemorrhage.
- Desensitizing inflamed folds with analgesics (painkillers) such as Tylenol® in order to phonate more comfortably desensitizes the singer and raises his risk of hurting the voice mechanism unawares.
- Aspirin and other anti-inflammatory analgesics such as ibuprofen and its relatives (Aleve®, Advil®, etc.) thin the blood and increase the risk of vocal fold hemorrhage if ingested during periods of heavy voice use. Even alcohol can interfere with blood clotting.

Who's susceptible?
- Singing and phonating with a varix induces swelling, making a hemorrhage more likely to occur. (See 10.4 Vocal Fold Varix.)
- Pregnant women have a greater risk of hemorrhaging with vocal strain.
- Women just prior to and at the onset of menstruation, especially if using aspirin products

How is it fixed?
- A hemorrhage can cause permanent damage to the vocal fold.
- One to three weeks of complete voice rest is often advised to resolve a hemorrhage and avoid possible scarring. The size of the blood vessel and the degree of leakage determine how serious the hemorrhage is.
- Five to six weeks of voice therapy is often recommended. Whether the hemorrhage was caused by a suppressed sneeze or poor singing technique will determine the therapy.
- Occasionally, and as a last resort, a hemorrhage mandates surgical intervention, in which laser **photocoagulation** should be used to eliminate the vessel(s) causing the leak.

10.4 VOCAL FOLD VARIX

What is it?
- A varix is a vascular (blood vessel) prominence and is a member of the varicose vein family. (See Figure 10.4.) A very tiny microvarix is commonly called a pepper speck.

How can you tell if you have it?
- Audibly: Blood is heavier than mucus, and a vocal fold with an enlarged capillary will have a greater weight than a normal fold. Two vocal folds of unequal

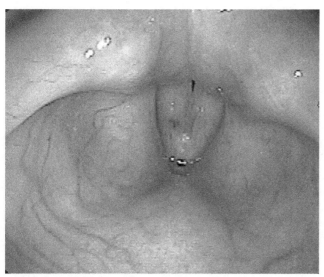

FIGURE 10.4 Vocal Fold Varix
Xenon lighting. Right vocal fold varicosity between 3 and 4. Folds are adducted and
phonating. Mutational chink suggests that this patient is a female.

weight will vibrate out of sync with each other, producing a distorted hoarse
sound. During phonation, a varix tends to swell. As the varix enlarges you may
hear a mild raspiness in the voice that starts after thirty to forty-five minutes of
vocalizing.

- Visibly: Enlarged or burst blood vessels can appear anywhere on the vocal fold,
  but often occur at the PMGC.
- Production variants: Loss of flexibility and range. Pop singers with varices
  often complain that the voice becomes tired and hoarse after the first set of
  songs in a concert and they are unable to perform the second set. With a few
  hours of voice rest a varix will decrease in size and the voice returns to the
  baseline level.

How do you get it?
- Over time with vocal abuse (excessive voice use) or vocal hyperfunction. Normal
  blood vessels enlarge during heavy voice use and extensive singing. Think of the
  varicose veins that tend to form in the ankles supporting the weight of a pregnant
  woman or near the knees of someone who habitually crosses her legs when sitting. Over time the walls of blood vessels will thin the more they are engorged.
  Eventually, blood will collect in the stretched-out areas of these channels and not
  flow through as efficiently.
- Dehydration, GERD, smoking, caffeine, allergies, and excessive alcohol consumption can irritate the folds and leave them in a less than optimal condition to
  vibrate, predisposing them to a varix formation.

- Desensitizing inflamed folds with analgesics such as Tylenol® in order to phonate more comfortably desensitizes the singer and raises his risk of hurting the voice mechanism unawares.

Note: Tylenol® is the analgesic of choice for singers in pain. Because it is acetaminophen rather than an anti-inflammatory, it doesn't thin the blood. However, singers must be careful when taking any analgesic because it will reduce their sensatory awareness within twenty minutes, including the ability to detect what is happening at the vocal fold level. Whenever perceptual feedback is dampened, singers run a higher risk of unintentionally straining the voice.

Who's susceptible?
- Heavy voice users
- Those who experience voice changes with PMS and continue to sing heavily during this time

How is it fixed?
- Voice conservation (including no singing) and occasionally voice rest are advised for possible self-resolution to avoid further irritation and bleeding.
- Occasionally, a varix mandates surgical intervention. The procedure is outpatient, and general anesthesia will not be necessary for a minor varix. A flexible scope is passed into the nose, through which a laser is used to photocoagulate the blood vessel.

10.5 VOCAL FOLD NODULES

What is it?
- Nodules are bilateral, symmetrical bumps that arise in the vocal folds' epithelium along the inner edge of the folds at the PMGC. (See Figures 10.5a and 10.5b.)Chronic friction over time slowly causes the affected area of the cover to thicken until nodules are formed. Nodules are similar to calluses on hands, developing from chronic overuse, and are the most common type of lesion found in singers.

How can you tell if you have it?
- Audibly: Hoarseness
- Visually: Early prenodular formation can be identified by stranding, frothy, or thickened mucus protectively collecting at the PMGC during phonation.

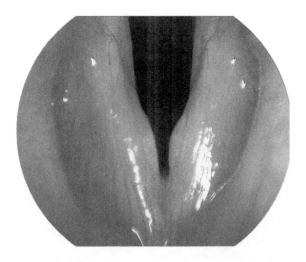

FIGURE 10.5a Vocal Fold Nodules (abducted)
Mature nodules from 3 to 4. Rough vocal fold edges and apparent bilateral vocal fold swelling and vascularity, suggesting chronic irritation.

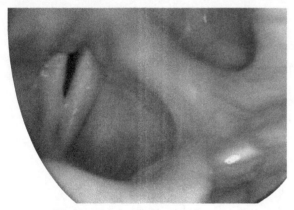

Figure 10.5b Vocal Fold Nodules (adducted)
Another pair of mature nodules showing hourglass appearance of vocal fold closure.

Nodules first appear as small, soft, edematous, and smooth outgrowths on the cover and along the free edge of each vocal fold. Over time, continued irritation from improper use enlarges and hardens the tissue, making nodules more fibrous, callus-like, and thus whiter looking. Once the nodules reach a critical size they interfere with closure, giving vocal fold closure an hourglass appearance. Occasionally nodules will appear closer to 3 than 4. Perhaps friction is greater a little bit closer to where the folds are more "pinned down" at the anterior commissure.

> Note: Nodules are always bilateral and symmetric, but some lesions may masquerade as nodules. For example, a cyst on one fold can cause reactive edema on the other, giving the illusion of nodules. It's safe to say that if two parallel lesions are not similar in size and shape, they are not nodules.

- Production variants: As the nodules get larger and stiffer with chronic bad vocal habits, phonation becomes increasingly effortful and the voice fatigues easily. Soft sounds become more difficult, vocal flexibility decreases, and range decreases—especially in the upper register—because the hardened tissue inhibits the folds' ability to elongate.

How do you get it?
- Dehydration, GERD, smoking, caffeine, allergies, and excessive alcohol consumption can irritate the folds and leave them in a less than optimal condition to vibrate and predisposed to nodule formation.
- Vocal abuse (speaking at too low a pitch, speaking too loudly, talking or singing too often or too long, poor singing technique, singing or speaking outside of your tessitura, or speaking in a constricted or harsh manner [e.g., rock musicians, athletic coaches])
- Even well-trained singers can develop nodules, but this is more often due to inappropriate use of their speaking voice, not their singing voice. Singers are often minimally educated regarding the appropriate use of the speaking voice. They don't necessarily think about applying what they've learned about healthy singing to their speaking voice. As a result, they can have habitual faulty speaking habits. (See Vocal Distortion-Not Glottal Fry, Speaking Pitch Too Low, and Hard Glottal Onsets in 3.9 Vocal Hazards.)

Who's susceptible?
- Those in heavy speaking professions (e.g., preachers, teachers, broadcasters)
- Untrained or poorly trained speakers and singers
- Adult females more than adult males, perhaps because they tend to speak in a lower than optimal tessitura or perhaps mutational chinks cause more stress to be placed on the anterior folds during phonation.

How is it fixed?
- Before treatment can be determined, videostroboscopy is used to assess vocal fold vibration around the nodules to gauge how hard or deep the nodules have become. Vibration present around the nodules indicates soft nodules that should respond well to therapy. Thick and nonvibrating nodules, especially those that harden tissue down to the superficial layer of the lamina propria, take longer to resolve if at all and may require surgery.

- Voice therapy is essential for those with any vocal fold nodules in order to retrain faulty vocal habits and prevent recurrence. Voice therapy resolves nodules in nearly 90% of the cases. The rate of resolution depends on the size and depth of the nodules and the ability of the individual to incorporate the changes required. On average it takes twelve to fourteen weeks for nodules to go away, and most singers can even return to singing before the nodules are completely gone.

- Some laryngologists now believe that lesions, whether nodules or polyps, never completely go away without surgical intervention. They believe that some tiny remnant of the pathology, perhaps invisible even with magnified exams, remains. This thinking is due to the number of patients with "resolved" nodules who revisit the clinic with lesions in the exact location of the previous injury. Perhaps repeat nodules are evidence of an anatomically "weak" or susceptible region in a patient's fold or perhaps the laryngologists are correct. Additional research will be needed to further investigate this topic.

- Surgery is rarely a good idea or a "quick fix" for vocal fold nodules. Surgery should be reserved for nodules that interfere with singing or speaking activities *and* don't resolve with voice therapy despite patient compliance. Because nodules form on the outermost layer of the epithelium and along the free vibrating edges of the vocal folds, removal involves cutting into the critical vibrating edge and can result in irreversible damage of the epithelium. Scar tissue will form during the healing process, possibly to the point of leaving the folds stiff and irregular, resulting in permanent hoarseness and limited range. (See Scarring in 12.1 Aspects of the Surgical Process That Concern Singers, and Vocal Fold Medial Edge Lesions in 12.3 Common Problems Where Surgery Could Affect the Voice Mechanism.)

- Occasionally, what appear to be nodules at the PMGC will be reabsorbed by the body with just a few days of voice rest. These are called *acute* nodules due to their quick formation and recovery time. Unlike prenodular swelling that occurs over a long period of time and takes a while to go away, acute nodules seem to develop in opera singers particularly and during a very short period of heavy hard performing. If voice rest is not heeded following the performance, the acute nodules can turn into a typical chronic nodule condition.

Note: Unless it's cancerous, a lesion that lies away from the vibrating edge of the vocal fold and isn't affecting the voice doesn't need to be removed. Many singers are able to live with small lesions and have very fine careers. I have a friend who has enjoyed a successful opera career, singing with a tiny pepper speck varix on her left vocal fold. The capillary protrusion is not close enough to the vibrating edge to interfere with her beautiful voice at all. And more than one country singer has visited the clinic who prefer to maintain small nodules on their folds for their trademark husky voice quality.

10.6 VOCAL FOLD CYST

What is it?
- A cyst is a unilateral (on only one vocal fold), very firm sac, deeply confined well under the epithelium. (See Figures 10.6a and 10.6b.) It forms in the superficial lamina propria due to a clogged duct or gland and rests on top of the vocal ligament. Depending on the type of duct or gland clogged, the firm sac may encapsulate blood, body serum, **squamous debris**, or mucus.

How can you tell if you have it?
- Audibly: Diplophonia, hoarseness
- Visibly: A smooth, round, raised area along the vibrating edge of the vocal fold, usually located at the PMGC. Its well-formed, nontransparent white membranous sac gives it the appearance of a white marble. Because it rests on the vocal fold ligament, vocal fold vibration is significantly inhibited or even prevented surrounding the cyst. The hardness of a cyst is irritating to the opposite vocal fold during vibration, and **reactive change** such as swelling and visible or broken capillaries can develop on the opposite fold. A protruding cyst on one fold paired with reactive swelling on the opposite fold can be mistaken for nodules, but keep in mind that nodules are symmetrical, whereas a cyst will most likely be larger than the swell it causes on the opposite fold. Therefore, asymmetric "nodules" should always raise the suspicion of a cyst. A cyst can remain unchanged, become denser, or even rupture over time.
- Production variants: Effortful vocalizing, easy vocal fatigue

How do you get it?
- A clogged duct (Usually the cause of the duct clogging is idiopathic; that is, it's unknown.)
- Anything that scars vocal fold tissue and prevents a duct from draining. Trauma to the vocal folds from a vocal misuse or abuse, reflux, smoking, infections (e.g., some type of laryngitis), or intubation (e.g., placement of a breathing tube for surgery) are examples.

Who's susceptible?
- Anyone

How is it fixed?
- It may be difficult to distinguish between a cyst, a polyp, and nodules. The initial treatment for all three conditions is voice therapy. Voice therapy can be used as a diagnostic tool whenever the lesion type is uncertain, and the pathology will be revealed over time. Once the true problem is identified, the treatment can be adjusted. A cyst is suspected when voice therapy helps to resolve reactive edema but little or no change occurs at the site of the lesion.

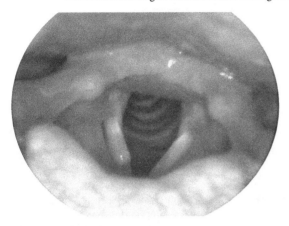

FIGURE 10.6a Vocal Fold Cyst
Right submucosal vocal fold cyst. Visible evidence of reactive change on the opposite fold is not clear from this picture.

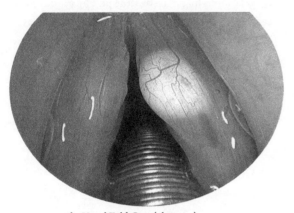

FIGURE 10.6b Vocal Fold Cyst (close-up)
Another right submucosal vocal fold cyst. Reactive change evident on left fold. Photo taken during microlaryngoscopy just prior to surgical removal. Patient is lying down, face up and is intubated, which accounts for the orientation of the picture.

- Although it never resolves a cyst, therapy should be used before surgery to reduce swelling surrounding the cyst and in the opposite fold. By reducing swelling, it's easier to define the size of the cyst and to enable more precise surgery by minimizing the amount of tissue requiring removal.
- Because cysts are often embedded so deeply in the vocal fold, multiple vocal fold layers are involved, requiring a more technically challenging surgery than removing a more superficial lesion such as a polyp. The surgeon should cut laterally alongside of, but away from the vibrating edge.

- Complete removal is required to resolve a cyst. Incomplete removal can result in the return of the cyst. Simply rupturing the cyst is not sufficient as a small shallow furrow or groove will develop in the surface and still limit vibration. (See 10.10 Sulcus Vergeture.)
- Cysts can be embedded into the vocal fold tissues as deep as the muscular layer and are likely to restrict vocal fold vibration to such a degree that over time the muscular layer atrophies. After surgery, much patience will be needed for postoperative voice therapy to get the underused muscles back in shape.

10.7 VOCAL FOLD POLYP

What is it?

- A polyp is a swelling anywhere in the epithelium and along the vibrating edge of the vocal fold. A polyp will often start nearer to cell layer 4 or 5 of the epithelium, also known as the basement membrane of the epithelium. A polyp can contain blood (hemorrhagic polyp), clear gelatinous material (**hyaline** polyp), blood vessels (angiomatous polyp), or scar tissue (fibrinous polyp). A polyp usually pops up on only one vocal fold (**unilateral** polyp) but can appear on both vocal folds as well (bilateral polyps).
- There are two types:
  - One type, called **sessile**, has a broad base and is simply a raised bump on the surface. (See Figure 10.7a.)
  - The other type is suspended, similar to a skin tag or mushroom, and is called **pedunculated** (literally "upon a stalk" or "pedestal"), as "ped-" means foot and this polyp sticks out as though it were a little foot. (See Figures 10.7b and 10.7c.)

How can you tell if you have it?

- Audibly: Hoarseness, diplophonia (A sessile polyp produces more consistent diplophonia than a pedunculated one. The pedunculated version has greater mobility and shifts unpredictably during vibration, producing sporadic diplophonia.)
- Visually: A bump often appearing at the PMGC that moves with vocal fold vibration. A fluid-filled polyp is soft and usually causes no irritation to the opposite fold. It may be recognized by its blister-like transparency revealing fluid that is clear (hyaline fluid) or dark red (blood), the latter of which is often fed by a visible blood vessel. A hard polyp, whether composed of dried blood or nontransparent fibrous tissue, often implies that the lesion has hardened with chronic irritation or age.
- Production variants: Patients can often recall the exact time they got a polyp due to a "pop" sensation in their throats when the polyp formed. (See 10.6 Vocal Fold Cyst.)

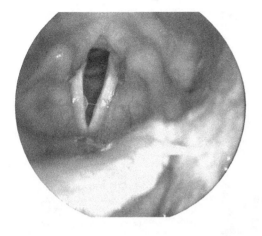

FIGURE 10.7a Sessile Polyp
Hyaline sessile polyp arising from right vocal
fold, area 3 to 4. Stranding mucus suggests
dehydration and some inflammation. Some
interarytenoid evidence of laryngopharyngeal
reflux.

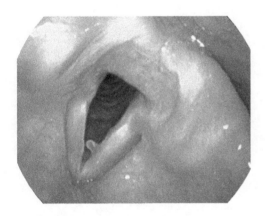

FIGURE 10.7b Pedunculated Polyp
Hyaline pedunculated polyp extending
from area 3 to 4 of left vocal fold.

How do you get it?

- Hyaline polyps most often occur from a cough or repeated yelling. (See Figures 10.7a and 10.7b.)
- Hemorrhagic polyps are the second most common lesion found in singers and are caused by a single more extreme vocal misuse, such as a loud hard scream, or a short-term overuse, like singing very loudly and high with a cold. (See Figure 10.7c.)

Who's susceptible?

- Those who use blood thinners are more susceptible to hemorrhaging and thus developing a polyp, as are those who sing during PMS and the common cold—both conditions that dilate the existing blood vessels of the vocal folds.

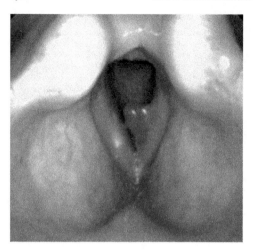

FIGURE 10.7C Hemorrhagic Polyp
Blood-filled polyp (pedunculated) arising
from 2 to 6 along the left vocal fold. Feeding
blood vessel not apparent. Some interarytenoid
evidence of laryngopharyngeal reflux.

- Those who yell at sporting events or during other situations where noise makes it hard to monitor your voice and especially during cold weather when the air tends to dry out the vocal folds
- Anyone using the voice with an altered vocal sensation. Consuming alcohol or the use of numbing throat lozenges can decrease the awareness of vocal sensation and mask an impending problem.

How is it fixed?
- Voice therapy is recommended first to see if it helps the polyp to resolve on its own. More often, however, polyps must be surgically removed.
- A pedunculated polyp is very unlikely to go away and usually requires surgical removal.
- Sessile polyps occasionally shrink and get reabsorbed by the body with therapy and voice conservation.
- When surgical intervention is necessary, the epithelial layer of the vocal fold can be gently lifted and the polyp surgically cut out. Because sessile polyps lie just under the surface of the folds' important medial edge, great care should be taken to cut the surface immediately alongside of but not on the vibrating edge of the vocal fold. Redundant tissue is carefully excised if the polyp is especially large and then the epithelium can be redraped, leaving the vibrating edge undisturbed. A polyp is not as deep as a cyst (very seldom will a polyp form from tissue as deep as the superficial lamina propria layer) but still requires operating within a crucial vibrating layer of the vocal fold. As with any surgery, the healing of the vocal fold and degree of scar formation determine the success of the outcome. (See Scarring in 12.1 Aspects of the Surgical Process That Concern Singers.)

- A laser may be needed to seal or **cauterize** blood vessels that feed a hemorrhagic polyp in order to minimize the risk of recurrence.
- A short period of complete voice rest (generally three to five days) is recommended after the operation to allow the wound to begin healing.
- Four to twelve weeks of voice therapy should follow the surgery to ensure improved vocal behaviors in order to prevent the return of the pathology and to monitor healing.

10.8 POLYPOID CORDITIS

What is it?
- Also known as polypoid degeneration, polypoid edema, or Reinke's edema, polypoid corditis is a thickened accumulation of the gel-like fluid in the superficial lamina propria layer of both vocal folds. (See Figure 10.8.)

How can you tell if you have it?
- Audibly: Extremely low speaking voice due to the increase in the vocal folds' mass, which causes the folds to vibrate more slowly (decreased frequency), resulting in a lower-sounding voice. This is more evident in the female speaking voice. The edema accompanying polypoid corditis may thicken the vocal folds to the extent that a female voice is even mistaken for a male voice on the phone.
- Visually: Polypoid corditis usually affects both folds fairly symmetrically, causing them to become thick and gelatinous with nondistinct polyp-like lumps. The entire lengths of the vocal folds are irregular and swollen and become discolored depending on the consistency of gel-like fluid. If the fluid is very thick, the folds will be gray, and if the fluid is thinner, they will be yellow. Unhealthy epithelium is thick and less transparent. In rare cases the vocal folds become very swollen and heavy to the point of getting sucked together on inhalation, making breathing difficult. The cover waves in an excessive and floppy manner due to the excess fluid retained inside.
- Production variants: Lack of flexibility, hoarseness, loss of upper range, difficulty breathing (thick heavy folds may obstruct airway and get sucked together on inhalation), inability to sustain a tone at a steady state

How do you get it?
- Commonly caused by first- or secondhand overexposure to vocally irritating inhalants (tobacco, marijuana, exhaust, chemicals, smoke, or asthma inhalers)
- Chronic gastric reflux
- Postnasal drip (sinusitis)
- Allergies
- Heavy, excessive voice use (more rare)

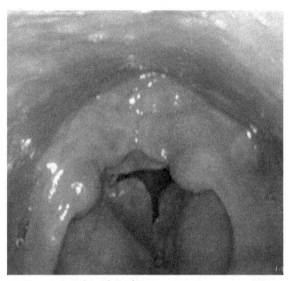

FIGURE 10.8 Polypoid Corditis
Vocal folds are abducted and airway is significantly obstructed. Discoloration and bilateral, nondistinct polypoid swelling affecting entire lengths of folds. Interarytenoid evidence of laryngopharyngeal reflux.

Note: Unfiltered cigarettes and marijuana deposit greater amounts of chemicals on the folds and are more likely to cause minor thermal irritation on the folds during inhalation than cigarettes that are filtered.

- Hypothyroidism, where low levels of thyroid hormone in the body cause fluid accumulation known as **myxedema** in the vocal folds
- **Angioedema**, a hereditary disorder due to an enzyme deficiency in the body. There is also an **idiopathic** form that is possibly triggered by allergies, chemical exposure, or trauma. Angioedema is the normal **lymphatic fluid** or serum in the body that leaves the circulation and diffuses into the tissues of the throat and larynx. This disorder involves the entire body and is not just limited to the vocal folds.

Who's susceptible?
- Professional voice users
- Allergic and asthmatic persons
- Smokers (This is not limited to heavy smokers. Polypoid corditis can develop even in those who smoke a few cigarettes a day. The susceptibility of individuals varies, where heavy smokers may never develop the polypoid changes and the "social smoker" will.)
- Car mechanics
- Chemical factory workers

How is it fixed?

- Depending on the severity of the pathology, treatment will vary.
- The response to any form of treatment is typically slow and may take months or even years to resolve.
- The disorder will come back as long as one continues to expose oneself to the irritant, so exposure to the irritant(s) must be reduced first.
- If only a little swelling is evident, voice therapy is recommended to reduce swelling.
- Corticosteroids may be used in some cases to mobilize the bound water, followed with careful, frequent monitoring of the lesion. It is common to use an oral steroid, such as prednisone, in addition to reflux medication.
- If the swelling is great and threatens the airway, surgery is a must and is done by cutting the vocal fold lateral to the midline to create a flap in the epithelium. The lining is then lifted, the thick fluid is sucked out, and the lining is redraped. This way, the vibrating edge of the vocal fold is left undisturbed.
- A laryngologist should determine whether to take a biopsy of the polypoid corditis to check for cancer. A biopsy is recommended if the folds are so stiff that their cover wave is reduced. Cancerous growth (i.e., malignancy) will often cause stiffness in the folds.
- If the polypoid corditis was caused from smoking and there is no cancer mandating immediate removal, many laryngologists will not remove the polypoid corditis until the person stops smoking.

10.9 VOCAL FOLD BOWING

What is it?

- This is also known as **myasthenia laryngis** and commonly called muscular atrophy. This condition refers to a decrease in muscle bulk resulting in a bowed appearance of the vocal folds. (See Figure 10.9.) The folds contact anteriorly and posteriorly but fail to close in the important middle portion of the vibratory true fold.
- The gap can increase slowly over time if more muscle bulk is lost.

How can you tell if you have it?

- Audibly: Breathiness, weak and overly quiet voice
- Visually: Vocal folds don't meet in the middle during phonation.

Note: Sometimes patients will have a very harsh, low voice if they are compensating with enough force to bring the false folds together for phonation. (See 10.15 Muscle Tension Dysphonia.)

- Production variants: Decreased vocal range (especially in lower register) with possible improvement when speaking slightly higher (due to the elongation of the folds), quick vocal fatigue due to extreme effort needed to phonate

How do you get it?
- Vocal fold bowing can occur from underuse or overuse.
- Vocal fold bowing can occur following vocal strain or injury (e.g., intubation).[1-4]
- Inevitable muscle deterioration with old age due to genetics and voice use (a symptom of presbylarynges or presbylarynx)
- Weakness due to virus or prolonged illness such as cancer
- Long-term use of inhaled corticosteroids
- Loss of nerve input to the vocal folds (See 10.16 Unilateral Vocal Fold Paralysis and Paresis.)
- Substantial weight loss
- Bowing at a young age suggests congenital lack of muscle development.

Who's susceptible?
- The elderly
- Those over fifty years old who take singing "breaks" for several weeks
- Overusers (e.g., retirees from high talking professions, such as retired professors, even if they're young)
- Underusers (e.g., singers who go on extended voice rest for more than two weeks)

How is it fixed?
- The regular use of the voice is important in maintaining muscle tone, just as exercise is important in maintaining all of the muscles in the body.
- The younger you are, the better your muscles can recover and gain strength with voice therapy and maintaining regular voice use.
- Once atrophy occurs in an older person, vocal strength is nearly impossible to regain. Regular use of the voice is necessary to maintain muscle tone, just as exercise is important in maintaining all muscles in the body. Consistent daily

[1] J. Stemple, J. Stanley, and L. Lee, "Objective Measures of Voice Production in Normal Subjects Following Prolonged Voice Use," *Journal of Voice* 9 (1995): 127–133.

[2] M. P. Gelfer, M. L. Andrews, and C. P. Schmidt, "Documenting Laryngeal Change Following Prolonged Loud Reading," *Journal of Voice* 10 (1996): 368–377.

[3] N. P. Solomon and M. S. DiMattia, "Effects of a Vocally Fatiguing Task and Systemic Hydration on Phonation Threshold Pressure," *Journal of Voice* 14 (2000): 341–362.

[4] N. P. Solomon et al., "Effects of a Vocally Fatiguing Task and Systemic Hydration on Men's Voices," *Journal of Voice* 17 (March 2003): 31–46.

vocalizing is important. Regular use will help maintain the voice without further muscle loss.

- Voice therapy will assist in exercising the folds in such a way as to tone the muscle and maximize closure. The therapy often involves training the voice to be hyperfunctional because extra effort is needed to gain closure for phonation.
- Surgically injecting Gelfoam®, Cymetra®, or fat into the folds can temporarily reshape the folds by bulking them up to achieve better closure for sound production. Injections are considered an option for singers only if they are having significant difficulty.
- Laryngeal reconstruction surgery (**laryngoplasty**) involves implanting a synthetic substance such as Silastic® or Gore-Tex® (polytetrafluoroethylene) between the inside of the thyroid cartilage wall and the muscular portion of the vocal fold

Note: Vocal fold bowing can also present in someone who has rheumatoid arthritis that affects the cricoarytenoid or cricothyroid joints. (See 5.9 Arthritis.) This type of bowing is usually mild and may not involve muscle loss at all but simply occur because of the way the vocal folds are situated. Cricothyroid joint stiffness may limit thyroid cartilage tilt so that the folds are unable to elongate well. Cricoarytenoid joint inflammation may disable the arytenoids from rocking back for very high pitches. Whether bowing stems from true atrophy or these positional reasons can be determined by having patients access their highest pitch range and observing joint motion and closure.

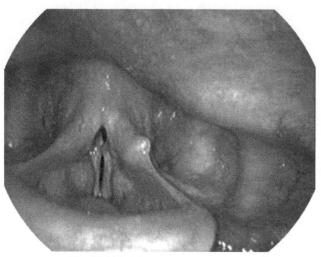

FIGURE 10.9 Vocal Fold Bowing
Adducted folds in the larynx of this older patient reveal that the folds are unable to close to the midline.

to push the entire fold closer to the midline. Implants are permanent and usually reserved for elderly patients with weak and breathy voices.

10.10 SULCUS VERGETURE

What is it?

- Also known as a sulcus vulgaris, a **sulcus vergeture** is an acquired dip in the vocal fold caused by the cover binding to the ligament underneath. (See Figure 10.10.)
- This is not to be confused with other types of vocal fold sulci (literally "grooves" in Latin):
  - Pseudo-sulcus: a.k.a. physiologic sulcus, infraglottic edema that mimics a sulcus vocalis but the superficial lamina propria is still there. This is sometimes seen with chronic dehydration or reflux, the latter of which can cause the lower portion of the vocal fold lip to stick out with swelling, making a groove-like appearance in the vocal fold.
  - Sulcus vocalis: A congenital pathology in which a deep groove in the vocal fold tissue dips down to the muscle, due to an absence of the superficial lamina propria, and impairs the voice.

How can you tell if you have it?

- Audibly: A "reedy" or "veiled" quality voice. The voice tends to be breathy with limited volume, and pitch may be slightly higher in a subconscious attempt to improve tone quality.
- Visually: A unilateral or bilateral tethered seam or invaginated dip of varying size, length, and depth in the vocal fold that runs laterally to the free edge of the fold. Extremely deep tethering may produce the appearance of a divided vocal fold. The typical exam will simply show bowing of the vocal fold and may be confused with a partial paralysis of the muscle. A sulcus is often not visible except on a videostroboscopy, which brings out the groove with the restricted cover wave. Folds that are tethered by a sulcus may only be able to meet along the bottom portion of the lip during phonation, producing only a partial cover wave.

Note: Physicians disagree on the use of the term "sulcus vocalis" and may generically refer to *any* dip or groove in the vocal folds as a "sulcus vocalis." We feel this is technically incorrect and distinguish "sulcus vocalis" from other sulci listed previously. The etiologies of sulci are controversial as well. There are many theories on whether particular sulci are acquired or congenital.

A. Giovanni, C. Chanteret, and A. Lagler. "Sulcus Vocalis: A Review." *European Archives Otorhinolaryngology Journal* 264, no. 4 (April 2007): 337–344.

- Production variants: Vocal fatigue, weak voice, reduced vocal range (especially in lower range), with possible improvement when speaking slightly higher due to the elongation of the folds. Impossible to sing

How do you get it?
- For the epithelium to adhere to the ligament underneath, the superficial lamina propria must be significantly damaged.
  - A preexisting vocal fold cyst ruptured
  - Intubation trauma

Who's susceptible?
- Anyone

How is it fixed?
- Voice therapy can improve and optimize the voice but will not completely resolve the problem.
- Voice therapy can help ease resulting secondary lesions and symptoms such as muscle tension dysphonia.
- Bulking vocal fold injections may compensate for the tethered area.
- Surgery is rarely effective. Because a sulcus is a deep lesion and tethers the vocal fold's outer layers (layers crucial to vibration) on or into the ligament, surgically separating these layers will simply cause them to heal together and cause retethering of the fold(s).
- At best, the patient will gain increased loudness from phonosurgery and therapy.

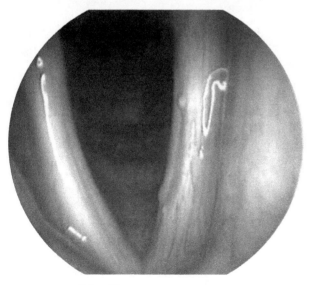

FIGURE 10.10 Sulcus Vergeture
Bilateral invagination of folds affecting medial vibrating edges.

10.11 LARYNGEAL GRANULOMA

What is it?

- A unilateral or bilateral grainy-looking (hence the name *granul*oma) buildup of raised red or gray tissue (depending on amount of blood flow to it) caused by chronic irritation to the mucosal lining of the arytenoids and/or the thin vocal fold epithelium covering the vocal processes. Layers of tissue form over layers of tissue. (See Figure 10.11.)

How can you tell if you have it?

- Audibly: Usually these lesions do not cause any audible voice symptoms because they typically appear around 7 to 9 on the vocal folds (the nonvibrating posterior portion of the vocal folds over the vocal process). Possible hoarseness, rough voice, breathiness, or diplophonia, if the granuloma is large enough to affect the phonation of the folds or if reflux is an aggravator
- Visually: Solid growths of red or pale gray redundant tissue along the vocal process of the arytenoids. The granuloma will develop a bilobed or saddle appearance due to the other true fold pressing against the mass. A portion of the granuloma will be above the edge of the fold and a portion below the edge. The point of contact is where the groove or indentation develops. The opposite fold can have a granuloma as well or often will show an ulcerated pit where the granuloma has rubbed against it during phonation. This picture is commonly called a "cup and saucer" or "ball and socket" due to its appearance. Granulomas that develop from intubation trauma are usually bilateral and similar in size. Arytenoids may overlap to compensate for lack of closure.
- Production variants: Frequent need to clear throat due to a lump feeling, morning hoarseness, easy vocal fatigue, voice weakens with use. This is one of the few vocal fold lesions that may cause pain at the vocal fold level. Referred pain may accompany this lesion and radiate up to the ear, mimicking an earache.

How do you get it?

- Granulomas are usually caused by some trauma to the vocal folds.
- They can be caused by or further aggravated by reflux.
- The back of the larynx is just in front of the esophagus, and the portion of the vocal fold over the vocal process (area 7 to 9) is thin, making it especially vulnerable to burns from regurgitated stomach acid. Even acid spilling onto the larynx once a day is sufficient enough to cause damage.
- Intubation trauma. Undergoing general anesthesia for surgery can result in intubation trauma to the posterior aspect of the larynx.

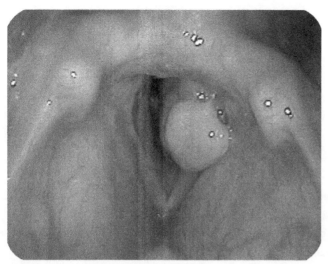

FIGURE 10.11 Laryngeal Granuloma
Large vocal fold granuloma, encompassing 4 to 9 on left vocal fold, extending subglottally into trachea and significantly narrowing airway. Apparent reactive change on right vocal fold.

- Unlike the rest of the vocal fold, the vocal process portion is epithelium and basement membrane over firm cartilage and is not padded by multiple layers of tissue. A vocal misuse (such as a loud yell) can cause the thin epithelial lining over the vocal process to tear and leave nothing to cushion the slamming together of the two vocal processes. This can lead to a low-grade infection and the development of granulated tissue.
- Vocal abuses that slam the arytenoids together (e.g., consistent too loud and too low phonation or using habitual hard glottal onsets)
- Chronic throat clearing or coughing

Who's susceptible?
- Anyone undergoing surgical intubation
- Women and some men who pitch their voices too low
- Teachers, preachers, lawyers, some singers who are vocally overactive
- Those using habitual hard glottal onsets and those with a chronic throat clear and/or cough
- Sufferers of GERD

How is it fixed?
- Train efficient voice production patterns with corrective voice therapy.
- Vigorous reflux treatment: Regulate diet and take prescribed reflux medication. Reflux management may take up to a year to resolve the granuloma.
- Oral steroids and a broad-spectrum antibiotic for two to three weeks may be suggested for a large and infected granuloma.

- Microlaryngeal surgery may be needed if these other methods fail to resolve the granuloma.
- Granulomas have a tendency to recur when treatment is not strictly adhered to or if some changes are not made in the vocal habits or diet.
- Intubation-related granuloma often resolves on its own.

10.12 LARYNGEAL CONTACT ULCERS

What is it?

- Laryngeal contact ulcers are unilateral or bilateral raw sores (ulcerated tissue) that form on the inner surface of the mucosa that covers the cartilaginous portion of the folds (a.k.a. the vocal process). (See Figure 10.12.) Some believe contact ulcers are a distinct disorder, but most physicians feel they are early-stage granulomas and that over time contact ulcers will enlarge and become granulomas.

How can you tell if you have it?

- Audibly: Possible hoarseness if contact ulcers are large enough. Frequently these lesions do not cause any audible voice symptoms because they typically appear on the vocal process (nonvibrating posterior portion of the vocal folds).
- Visually: Indentations or ulcerations appear on the posterior aspect of the vocal folds along the vocal processes of the arytenoids.
- Production variants: Incessant need to clear throat due to a lump feeling, morning hoarseness, vocal fatigue, and voice weakening with use. Like granulomas, contact ulcers are one of the few voice disorders that can cause pain at the vocal fold level.

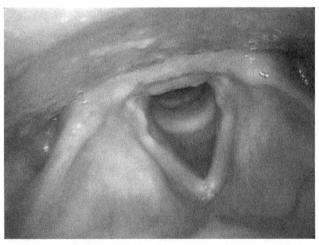

FIGURE 10.12 Laryngeal Contact Ulcers
Bilateral sores along the vocal processes (7 to 9) of the vocal folds.

Note: When viewing your exam pictures or video with the laryngologist, be careful to check for growths during abduction, as well as adduction and phonation. Contact ulcers and granulomas may not be readily visible as they can slip out of view when the folds come together for phonation.

How do you get it?
- Almost always associated with chronic reflux
- Surgical intubation
- Frequent throat clearing or coughing
- Vocal abuses that slam the arytenoids together (e.g., consistent too loud and too low phonation or using habitual hard glottal onsets)
- Loud low phonation

Who's susceptible?
- Anyone undergoing surgical intubation
- Women and some men who pitch their voices too low
- Teachers, preachers, lawyers, some singers who are vocally overactive
- Those using a habitual hard glottal onset
- Sufferers of GERD

How is it fixed?
- Ulcers need a minimum of six weeks of voice conservation to heal.
- Corrective behavioral voice therapy if the cause is related to vocal abuse
- Vigorous treatment of reflux
- Intubation-related contact ulcers often resolve on their own.

10.13 LARYNGEAL WEB

What is it?
- A **laryngeal web** is a band of tissue, usually small and thin, that connects the true folds at their anterior commissure. Most often vocal fold webbing extends from the anterior commissure up to the PMGC. (See Figures 10.13a and 10.13b.)

How can you tell if you have it?
- Audibly: Varies depending on length and width of web. Usually tight, high-pitched phonation. Can be similar to a sulcus' "reedy" or "veiled" quality voice. The voice tends to be breathy because the folds don't adduct very well

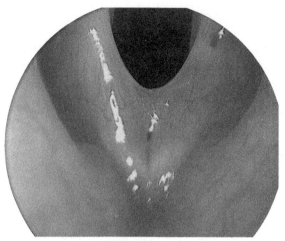

FIGURE 10.13a Laryngeal Web
Close-up of a vocal fold web affecting anterior commissure 1 to 2.

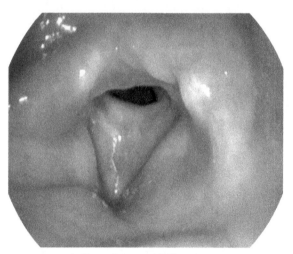

FIGURE 10.13b Severe Laryngeal Web
Vocal folds are abducted. A large vocal fold web spans the glottis and binds the full length of the folds. The airway is significantly obstructed.

just above the web. Volume is limited due to anterior tethering, and the voice is pitched slightly higher (due to a shorter vibrating portion of the folds and a subconscious attempt to improve tone quality).

- Visually: Like a webbed animal's foot, a laryngeal web is a **concave**, semilunar tethered band of tissue between the vocal folds at the anterior commissure. The web's tissue is similar in color to the vocal folds and is seen adjoining the two folds where they join in front.

- Production variants: Webbing at the vocal fold level can limit vocal fold vibration, and if the web extends past the PMGC, the folds may not even be able to adduct. In rare cases, a laryngeal web may narrow the airway (stenosis) to the point of obstructing and restricting airflow. Someone with a tiny "microweb" may never know they have one. Although it is rare, a microweb can increase the strain on the remaining vibratory portions of the vocal folds to the point that nodules develop.

How do you get it?
- Webs most commonly form during the healing of bilateral wounds near the anterior commissure. Whether due to bilateral surgical incision (e.g., overly aggressive removal of nodules) or bilateral intubation trauma to the folds, the wound can heal together, bonding tissues across the glottis.

Who's susceptible?
- Anyone undergoing surgical intubation
- Anyone undergoing laryngeal surgery
- Anyone undergoing radiation to the neck area (treatment for glottal or supraglottal carcinoma)

How is it fixed?
- Surgical separation of vocal folds, although the outcome may be poor. Because the separation leaves the folds with bilateral open wounds at the anterior commissure, the folds often heal back together the same way.

Note: Webbing can also be congenital, in which the vocal folds never completely separated during embryogenesis (i.e., development in the womb). Congenital webbing tends to occur just *below* the anterior commissure and rarely affects sound quality or vibration. People with congenital webbing, however, are more likely to develop nodules and may not know they have a web until they are evaluated and diagnosed with nodules. It's hard to say why congenital webbing predisposes people to nodules, but it likely has something to do with the web creating more stress during vibration in the PMGC region above.

Note: Webbing can also occur in the trachea from an intubation trauma to the windpipe. This is called tracheal stenosis.

10.14 LARYNGEAL PAPILLOMA

What is it?

- Papillomatosis is caused by a virus, the human **papilloma** virus (**HPV**),[5] which runs in the herpetic family (in other words, a type of herpes) and produces a wart-like growth that can recur and spread (in which case it's called *recurrent laryngeal papilloma*). (See Figure 10.14.) If it spreads to the lungs, it can be life threatening. There are twenty-three varieties of this virus, of which #6 and #11 are the subtypes associated with the larynx.

How can you tell if you have it?

- Audibly: The growths weigh down the folds, often allowing air to escape and resulting in hoarseness.
- Visually: Laryngeal wart-like growths that develop on the epithelium that lines the vocal folds. They look like cauliflower or fish eggs and may be white or reddish depending on the presence of feeding blood vessels.
- Production variants: The size of the growths and the rate at which they multiply can restrict airways and obstruct airflow, resulting in difficulty breathing. Breathing difficulty is more common in pediatric patients due to smaller airways being affected.

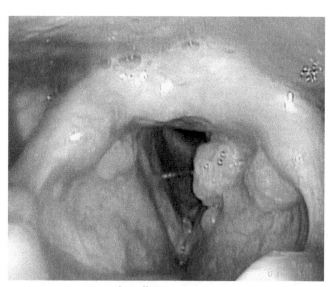

FIGURE 10.14 Laryngeal Papilloma

Large papilloma affecting left vocal fold 4 to 9, extending into ventricle and onto posterior portion of the left false fold surface. Papilloma is also apparent in left ventricle, just anterior to large papilloma. Another large papilloma just superior and lateral to the left false fold arises from the laryngeal vestibule wall. More papilloma is visible on the superior and posterior surface of the right false fold and from 1 to 2 along the right vocal fold's medial edge, obstructing anterior commissure. Stranding mucus due to inflammation.

---

[5] Also seen as two words, "human papillomavirus."

Note: A person can be infected with the human papilloma virus without any physical signs. The virus can exist in the body and never produce any wart-like growths.

How do you get it?
- HPV is an airborne infection contracted from another infected individual. Nearly everyone is exposed to the virus, but most people are able to fight off the virus and never develop laryngeal papilloma.
- Some research shows it can be transmitted in the birth canal during delivery, if the mother is infected.
- Engaging in oral sex with an infected individual
- Passing through an infected birth canal during delivery
- A preexisting viral component of papilloma may lie dormant in the body. If susceptible tissue is disrupted during a surgery, the virus may be activated.

Who's susceptible?
- Anyone, although infants and children under six years old are more susceptible to chronic papilloma

How is it fixed?
- Active papilloma requires surgery. The pathology will not resolve on its own.
- Papillomas are removed surgically with a laser or an instrument called a **microdebrider**. The microdebrider sucks in and chews up papillomas.
- Laser vaporization is the most effective way to destroy papilloma and takes away less tissue than using a surgical knife to cut it away. When a laser is used to vaporize papilloma, special facemasks must be worn throughout surgery that filter out the papilloma virus and ensure that live viral particles are not transmitted through laser smoke (a.k.a. "laser plumes") to others in the operating room.
- The primary reason to remove the papilloma is to improve vocal quality and maintain an open airway.
- Care is taken to minimize scar tissue formation to ensure optimum voice quality. This is a superficial disease, and it is not necessary to cut deeply into the folds. If the papilloma presents along the anterior aspect of the folds, the surgeon should take care to operate on one vocal fold at a time to prevent a laryngeal web from forming during healing.
- *Recurrent* laryngeal papilloma is a lifelong condition and a form of the virus that necessitates multiple surgeries as frequently as every few months, though typically every twelve to eighteen months, to improve the sound of the voice. More frequent removal of papilloma along the vocal folds may eventually cause excessive scarring, prohibiting complete vocal fold closure. If while in remission the folds are directly

disturbed (e.g., by an intubation—not by a hard cough), the papilloma can flare up. Papilloma can go into remission and stay dormant only to flare up without warning thus even a tiny inactive papilloma that is not interfering with the voice must be monitored closely. Damage caused by multiple surgeries may require corrective surgery. In extreme cases, counteractive medialization surgery may be performed with great caution to bulk up the vocal folds. Rarely must a total **laryngectomy** be performed. Even after a total laryngectomy, however, the laryngeal warts are likely to recur in the trachea—days or even ten to thirty years later.

- Several antiviral medications can be used. Future advancements include the use of a vaccine for HPV that is already available for experimental use.

10.15 MUSCLE TENSION DYSPHONIA

What is it?

- Muscle tension dysphonia (MTD) is any degree of vocal hyperfunction that results in inefficient phonation. In severe cases, false fold phonation can result (also known as "ventricular dysphonia," "false fold phonation," or "dysphonia plicae ventricularis"). MTD is one of the more common vocal disorders seen in singers. (See Figure 10.15.)

How can you tell if you have it?

- Audibly: Usually a tight, pressed sound. If vocal fold constriction is severe, the false folds may be squeezed together enough to touch and phonation can occur.

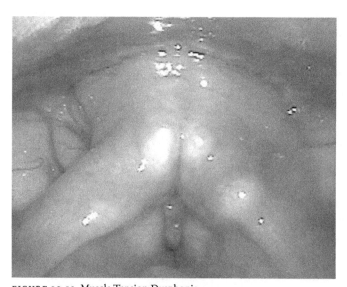

FIGURE 10.15 Muscle Tension Dysphonia
The entire laryngeal vestibule is squeezing inward during phonation, placing a great deal of constriction on the true vocal folds. Although not touching, the false folds are considerably approximated.

False folds are heavier and thus vibrate at a lower frequency. Their lack of fine muscle control results in the inability to fluctuate the frequency of their vibration. This produces a low-pitched, monotonous, and coarse sound. Extreme MTD may cause diplophonia due to the dual source of true and false fold vibrations vibrating out of phase with each other.

Note: Because the false folds have muscular properties, they can approximate and, with significant effort and continuous muscle tension, develop vibration. Over time, we've even observed consistently practiced false fold phonation develop a regular periodic vibration and a mucosal wave. (Here the term "mucosal wave" is used accurately, because the false folds *are* covered in mucosa.) False fold phonation is considered pathologic in healthy patients and is a result of extreme MTD. However, false fold phonation can actually become an acceptable substitute voice in patients who are compensating for irreversible damage to the true vocal folds, such as folds stiff with scarring from repeat vocal fold cancer or papilloma surgeries.

- Visually: Larger than normal mutational chink in females, incomplete posterior closure in males. An anterior gap may be noted as well. Slight approximation to severe compression of the false folds, which can obstruct the view of the true folds. Slight to severe anterior to posterior compression of the epiglottis to the arytenoids, and possibly constricted aryepiglottic sphincter
- Production variants: Vocal fatigue, laryngeal muscle fatigue, and anterior neck ache discomfort

---

Note: MTD is occasionally diagnosed when no other pathology accounts for the person's description of the problem and when "ache" or "vocal fatigue" is present.

How do you get it?

- MTD often develops to compensate for and overcome a less than optimum vibratory pattern, whether the culprit is postsurgery swelling, reflux-related swelling, vocal fold paralysis, or disruptive lesions such as nodules or a cyst.
- MTD can also develop in individuals with asthma, emphysema, or bronchitis who have less airflow available to drive the voice. To increase the subglottal pressure enough to initiate vocal fold vibration, the folds must increase the compressive forces between the folds. This activity requires an increase in sustained

muscle contraction. The increased muscle activity causes a "squeezed" voice and the extra muscle effort leads to rapid vocal fatigue. Over time the individual cannot sustain the effort required to continue with phonation.
- Stress and anxiety can also cause some people to tighten at the laryngeal level, in which case the MTD may be referred to as functional dysphonia.

Who's susceptible?
- Those who "oversing," sing with a compromised instrument (such as one affected by a cold), or sing to compensate for and cover up a vocal pathology (such as a polyp or nodules)
- Singers who sing with poor singing technique
- Singers who experience a "tired" voice and need to "tweak" the voice in order to push through the performance
- Those with asthma, emphysema, or bronchitis who compensate for a lack of airflow by increasing laryngeal muscle activity
- Sufferers of other vocal pathologies (such as papilloma or large lesions) who are compensating for poor approximation

How is it fixed?
- It is important to establish the etiology of the MTD and correct the cause and not just treat the symptom. A full-picture assessment of the patient is crucial (e.g., a patient may have a hidden culprit such as hypernasality from a **velum** that is too low and may push the voice to sound louder).
- If hyperactive laryngeal musculature becomes habitual, a more balanced muscle activity can be achieved with voice therapy.
- Laryngeal massage may also help ease MTD and can be combined with corrective voice therapy.

Note: Occasionally stress may cause laryngeal muscles to be held so tightly that *no* voice can be produced. This type of muscle tension disorder is called functional aphonia.

10.16 UNILATERAL VOCAL FOLD PARALYSIS AND PARESIS

What is it?
- A vocal fold paralysis (a.k.a. complete vocal fold paralysis) is a condition in which one (unilateral) or both (bilateral) of the true vocal folds are completely

immobile due to a total lack of nerve input to the larynx. It is also classified as **central** if due to a central nervous system (brain) disorder or **peripheral** if due to disorders of the vagus nerve or one of its branches (recurrent laryngeal nerve or superior laryngeal nerve). A unilateral paralysis is the most common type encountered and is the type discussed here. (See Figures 10.16a and 10.16b.)

- A vocal fold paresis (a.k.a. partial vocal fold paralysis) is when one or both vocal folds have limited motion due to weakened nerve input to the larynx. A unilateral paresis is the most common type and is discussed here.

Note: Bilateral paralyses in which both folds are frozen in an adducted, abducted, or anywhere in between position are fortunately rare and therefore not included here.

How can you tell if you have it?
- Audibly:
  - An affected superior laryngeal nerve (SLN) involving the external branch will prevent the folds from ascending in pitch. An affected SLN involving the internal branch is often harder to detect. It tends to cause subtle symptoms, such as frequent throat clearing and sudden coughing fits.
  - Significant voice changes occur, however, when the recurrent laryngeal nerve (RLN) is affected. The quality of the voice will depend on the ability of the "normal" fold to meet the paralyzed fold. If the fold is paralyzed in a median position (in the middle of the glottis), the voice can be nearly normal with some loss of high and low notes. When the fold is in a paramedian position (near the middle of the glottis), the voice is usually breathy with limited dynamic range. When the fold is frozen in a lateral position (abducted to the side), the voice is a very weak, breathy whisper.
  - With an RLN paresis, voicing is usually possible with increased effort. Such effort results in rapid vocal fatigue and a strained quality to the sound.
- Visually:
  - A damaged external SLN will leave folds unable to elongate for higher pitches.
  - A damaged RLN will paralyze a fold in a median, paramedian, or lateral position. The frozen fold will eventually thin due to a loss of muscle tone. The mobile fold will try to reach the paralyzed fold to phonate and will succeed when the frozen fold is in a median or paramedian position. Closure will be incomplete, however, and result in a bowed appearance to some degree. The mobile fold will not be capable of crossing to meet a fold frozen in a lateral position.
  - When a *paresis* is caused by an RLN weakness, the affected vocal fold will not abduct or adduct as rapidly. Under videostroboscopy the partially paralyzed fold may have a cover wave but may vibrate out of phase with the healthy fold due to a difference in muscle tone.

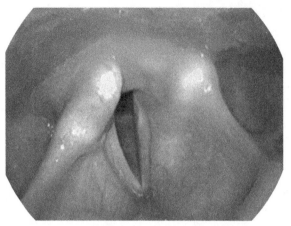

FIGURE 10.16a Unilateral Vocal Fold Paralysis (abducted)
Although difficult to determine the side of paralysis in a still picture, the right vocal fold pictured here is shorter and slightly bowed on abduction, suggesting that it is the affected fold. The left fold looks somewhat strained, and its color suggests inflammation.

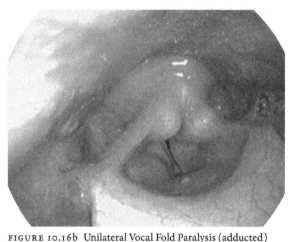

FIGURE 10.16b Unilateral Vocal Fold Paralysis (adducted)
This adducted view of the same vocal folds helps to confirm the prediction in the caption of Figure 10.16a that this is a right vocal fold paralysis. The left side is working so hard to adduct to the frozen right side that the false fold has actually adducted beyond the median and completely obscured the true fold underneath it. The left true fold remains as it appeared in abduction, but the left false fold seems less affected and is enervated enough to attempt some medialization.

- Production variants: Persistent vocal difficulty with very little day-to-day variation
  - A damaged internal branch of the SLN will decrease laryngeal sensitivity and the ability to clear or swallow. This desensitivity can lead to choking, aspirating, or producing unintentional "gurgly" sounds during phonation due to pooling liquid around folds. The voice will struggle to sustain its highest

pitches (due to incomplete closure). The voice will only be able to ascend so high in pitch before it hits a ceiling and simply cannot go any higher.

- A damaged RLN will leave most patients with a lump feeling in the throat and swallowing difficulty. The more lateral the fold's paralysis is, the quicker the vocal fatigue due to effortful approximation for phonation. A fold paralyzed in a lateral configuration is difficult to compensate for and usually results in choking (due to aspiration) when eating because the trachea is always substantially exposed.
- A paresis due to a damaged RLN will make it impossible to sustain a steady tone due to the two sides vibrating at an unsynchronized rate.

> Note: Symptoms that come and go with periods of a normal voice are not typical for a nerve disorder.

How do you get it?
- Disruption to the RLN, SLN, or higher up on the vagal nerve, which would affect both the RLN and the SLN
  - The most common cause of a unilateral paralysis is a surgical procedure mishap (iatrogenic). Unilateral paralysis is more common on the left side because the RLN has a longer course into the chest and can be damaged from any chest/ heart procedure. The RLN is commonly damaged (up to 10% of the time) in patients having chest/heart surgery, thyroid surgery, lung surgery, esophageal surgery, and cervical disc surgery. The RLN can also be easily damaged when too large a breathing tube (**endotracheal tube** [**ETT**]) is inserted for general anesthesia. The RLN enters the larynx behind the cricothyroid joint and travels up between the arytenoid and the inside of the thyroid cartilage wall. Because the placement of any endotracheal tube moves the arytenoids to some degree, this nerve is susceptible to getting pinched and temporarily or permanently damaged, especially if the tube used is larger than necessary.
  - Often the cause of a vocal fold paralysis is never identified (idiopathic) and thought to be viral induced.
- The causes of a paresis are the same as a complete paralysis with the addition of a stroke. A cerebral vascular accident (stroke) will rarely cause a paralysis but can cause a unilateral vocal fold weakness.

Who's susceptible?
- Anyone undergoing thoracic, head, or neck surgery or any procedure involving general anesthesia
- Anyone is susceptible to viral infections triggering paralysis.

How is it fixed?

- First. it is important to determine whether the complete paralysis will resolve on its own. A normal waiting period is nine to twelve months to allow the nerve to recover. During this waiting period, professional voice users may want to consider an in-office laryngoplasty procedure in which an implant material such as Cymetra® or Radiesse® is injected directly into the vocal folds. The injection is done through the mouth with a curved needle or through the neck (cricothyroid membrane) with a short needle to beef up the folds to temporarily improve phonation. Improvement is immediate and a sufficient amount is determined by having the patient talk in between doses and monitoring the folds via nasendoscopy throughout.
- Roughly half of the cases of vocal fold paralysis will resolve over time. Recovery is variable and can be complete or incomplete. Unless complete normal regeneration occurs, a singer will be left with a permanent change in the voice. Fine motor control may never return and leave vocal range and stamina limited.
- Early initiation of voice therapy is always a good idea.
- If the paralysis is identified early and a viral etiology is suspected, then antiviral medication and oral corticosteroids can help quicken recovery.
- If the etiology is iatrogenic, then oral corticosteroids alone are usually prescribed.
- Early surgical intervention is reserved for those who depend on the voice for their profession. Surgery will help the speaking voice but is unlikely to restore the singing voice back to a performance level.
- For a paralysis that doesn't resolve, treatment depends on the position of the vocal fold and the functioning of the larynx.
  - If the fold is frozen in a position near the middle of the glottis (i.e., a paramedian position), treatment may not be needed aside from voice therapy to help optimize the voice.
  - A fold in a paramedian position may benefit from surgical injections of silicon, Gelfoam,® or fat to plump it up so the opposite fold may vibrate against it.

Note: Fat is taken by liposuction, usually from the belly, and must be overinjected because some will be reabsorbed by the body.

- A laryngeal reconstruction surgery with medialization using an implant may help. This medialization procedure involves surgically creating an opening into the thyroid cartilage and placing an implantable material (such as a soft wedge of Gore-Tex® or thyroid cartilage) into the lateral thyroarytenoid region just inside the thyroid cartilage that pushes the muscle and medial vibrating edge to the midline. This procedure is a permanent fix and more precise than the injection procedures. The injections are best reserved for patients with a small gap who do not require much additional bulk.

- When the fold is in a lateral position, the medialization procedure described previously is required to restore the voice.

Note: Silastic® and Teflon® are no longer popular substances for medialization procedures. Silastic, a form of silicon, is difficult to place on implantation. Teflon® is a very hard synthetic substance that tends to migrate from position. Its stiffness can hinder the vocal fold's vibratory pattern and cause long-term irritation.

- The success of recovery from a paresis is greater than from a complete paralysis and usually takes only two to three months to resolve. Treatment protocols and surgical procedures are basically the same as with a complete paralysis, with the exception that medialization surgery is infrequently done or needed to correct bowing.

10.17 ARYTENOID DISLOCATION

Although this is not a common injury, we felt it important to include.

What is it?

- When an arytenoid cartilage completely separates from the cricoarytenoid joint space to the point of tearing the anterior and/or posterior cricoarytenoid ligaments (usually both)

Note: There is also an injury called arytenoid subluxation (AS) in which an arytenoid slides partially out of position within the joint. This can occur with extreme power lifting for which a very strong Valsalva is required—not simply picking up a couch—and may cause a click sensation at the time of the displacement and its resolve. Some research suggests that those with diabetes mellitus, chronic renal failure, rheumatoid arthritis, and long-term corticosteroid use may be more susceptible to AS.

Joshua Schindler and Yvette Leslie. "Arytenoid Dislocation." *edicine* from *WebMD,* updated January 7, 2010. http://emedicine.medscape.com/article/866464-overview.

How can you tell if you have it?
- Audibly: Severe hoarseness, possibly no voice at all
- Visually: Arytenoid looks out of place, red and swollen, asymmetrical arytenoids
- Production variants: Instant pain with possible pop sensation at the time of the incident, clicking feeling, every swallow and effort to talk hurts severely

How do you get it?
- Acute, sudden onset due to a mechanical trauma:
  - Rough intubation or extubation
  - Endotracheal tube size too large
  - Poor placement of a laryngoscope
  - Poor placement of nasogastric tube used to pump stomach
  - Poor placement of feeding tube if one can't swallow

Who's susceptible?
- Anyone

How is it fixed?
- A dislocated arytenoid will not spontaneously resolve on its own and mandates immediate surgery with general anesthesia. A surgical probe is needed to get behind and relocate the displaced cartilage within forty-eight hours of the trauma or the joint will fuse out of place, permanently leaving the patient with something similar to a paralyzed vocal fold.

10.18 LARYNGEAL SICCA

What is it?
- Laryngeal dryness

How can you tell if you have it?
- Audibly: Chronic cough
- Visually: Vocal folds appear dehydrated, thick mucus prevalent, cover wave decreased
- Production variants: Possible dry mouth, dry throat, desire to cough while singing (although some people grow accustomed to effects of dehydration and don't notice it), thick mucus, loss of freedom to the voice, vocal onset difficulty (harder to initiate phonation)

How do you get it?
- Side effect of medication (e.g., antihistamines, decongestants, proton pump inhibitors for reflux)

- A chronic autoimmune disorder called **Sjögren's** (SHOW-grinz) **syndrome** in which white blood cells attack mucous glands

Who's susceptible?

- Anyone

How is it fixed?

- If the sicca is due to a side effect, stop taking the medication that is causing the sicca and substantially increase your water intake.
- If an autoimmune disorder is the cause, a medication called a sialagogue can help to decrease symptoms by increasing mucus. (See 11.13 Mucolytics.)

Note: We have known a few voice teachers who assume a student's thick mucus is due to reflux and casually suggest a reflux medication. The reflux medication then exacerbates the symptoms, worsening the dryness and provoking more thick mucus. Be sure to get a medical diagnosis before self-medicating.

10.19 ESSENTIAL VOCAL TREMOR

What is it?

- An essential tremor is a neurological disorder that causes trembling of a body part. Essential vocal tremor means that it involves the voice. In most cases, a tremor begins gradually, usually in the hands or head and sometimes progressing to the voice. Essential means that it's not associated with other diseases.

How can you tell if you have it?

- Audibly: An essential tremor in the voice will sound like a slow wobble. You can't mask the wobble by putting a vibrato on it because even the resonating cavities will have the tremor.
- Visually: Laryngeal structures will shake or wobble in a rhythmic pattern during voicing.
- Production variants: The tremor worsens with caffeine, stress, lack of sleep, and exposure to extreme temperatures.

How do you get it?

- Comes on later in life, usually in the fifties or sixties
- Idiomatic but seems to be genetic

Who's susceptible?
- Anyone. About 50% are hereditary.

How is it fixed?
- It's not fixed. It's controlled. Medications usually help with hands and head but not voice.
- Some notice that it gets better after one glass of alcohol.
- **BOTOX**® injections into the vocal fold can help diminish the voice wobble with varying degrees of success. Because the essential tremor can affect so many muscles (oral, laryngeal, and neck) that are contributing to the wobble, multiple injection sites to correct a wobble may leave the patient very weak with minimal improvement.
- Voice therapy can benefit those who develop too much tension in the voice out of efforts to try to control the wobble.

11

Vocally Hazardous Drugs

YOU NEED TO be informed about drugs that pose potential dangers to your voice. If you are not familiar with a medication, do not hesitate to ask a physician about potential side effects. However, because the majority of physicians are not aware of how medications can affect the voice, it is best if you also investigate medicationsyourself. By educating yourself, you will be able to collaborate with the physician in selecting a singer-friendly antidote. Medications do change over time. To learn more about a medication or to find out about a medication not listed in this chapter, consult the annually published *Physicians' Desk Reference* (PDR) at your public library to find all up-to-date prescription medications, their side effects, and their potential complications.A good Internet resource is the National Library of Medicine at http://www.nlm.nih.gov. (This is the primary source Dr. Arick Forrest used to check the side effects listed in this chapter.) The National Center for Voice and Speech also offers an online chart of medications called "Check Your Meds: How Do They Affect Your Voice?" at http://www.ncvs.org/rx.html.

This chapter is not promoting that you self-medicate. Self-medication may prove harmful. This chapter is intended to help you to be well informed of many over-the-counter (OTC) and prescription (Rx) medications and their effects on the voice so that you can consult and work with your physician to get the best treatment.

Some general advice before taking any medication:

- Always be aware of medications that can cause dry mouth, dizziness, or sedation. These medications can adversely affect your performance.
- As a general rule, a singer should not use any medication unless absolutely necessary.

- Do a "trial" period with the medication. Make sure that the first time you try the medication is not right before a performance. Try the medication on a nonperforming day, but definitely try singing while you are on the medication. (Most oral medications begin to take effect thirty to forty-five minutes after ingesting.)
- There will be times when a trial period is not possible. Under these circumstances you need to decide how important the performance is and whether it's worth not being at your full potential or risking vocal injury. (For example, singing with an upper respiratory infection can result in vocal fold injury that may take weeks or even months to resolve. On rare occasions this can also require surgery for correction!) The degree of difficulty of the performance is a factor in the decision process.
- Every individual reacts differently to medication, and the dosing to achieve the desired effect can vary.

Because drugs can be referred to by their generic or chemical names, and because new medications come out all the time, we have decided to help you understand how *classes* of medications can adversely affect the voice. Although not exhaustive, this chapter groups common medications into classes, with an emphasis on hazardous agents. A brand name is included in parenthesis after each drug's generic chemical name. If you have questions about a brand name not mentioned in this book, please refer instead to the generic name on the box or bottle and check the index at the back of the book.

11.1 ALLERGY AND COLD MEDICATIONS

Most of the medications used for colds or allergies are drying and may thicken your secretions. This may be a desired effect when a singer has abundant secretions from a cold or allergic reaction. An important point to remember is that the saliva and mucus we produce is protective for the throat and larynx. The production of nasal, oral, and laryngeal secretions are all tied together. The perception of "excess" mucus can be due to overproduction of mucus or drainage that is too thick. A healthy body produces roughly a quart of mucus each day. As long as mucosal secretions are thin, they are swallowed and are not perceived as being excessive.

> Note: There are two components or ingredients that form mucus and determine whether mucus is thick or thin. One of the components is thin and watery and the other is a protective and lubricating component called mucin. Each component is produced in numerous tiny glands and deposited into pipe-like ducts to be combined. The final mixed product—mucus—is secreted out of the ducts into a cavity, such as the larynx or nose. The balance between the two components in the final mixture is critical for easy singing.

Many medications decrease the thin watery component in mucus without decreasing the stickier lubricating component, leaving the singer with a dry mouth that feels "gummy" or sticky. Singers often take medications to dry nasal drainage, but these are notorious for also decreasing the production of oral and laryngeal secretions. The unbalanced viscous mucus secreted at the laryngeal level can collect on the vocal folds and be very disruptive when trying to phonate. Thick mucus on the folds will produce a heavy feeling and interrupt phonation. The drying effect of the medication will cause epithelial mucus secretions to become viscous as well, resulting in more friction between the vocal folds during phonation, provoking swelling and quick vocal fatigue. The majority of these medications are also sedating. A good idea is to start with a pediatric dose and slowly raise or **titrate** the dosage until the desired effect is reached. Over-the-counter preparations generally use pseudoephedrine and Benadryl® as the most common ingredients. Benadryl® should be avoided, but pseudoephedrine in small doses (15 mg) is acceptable and easier to control. Be cautious of medications containing nonsteroidal anti-inflammatory medications (such as ibuprofen), as these are blood thinners. With an upper respiratory infection (e.g., a cold), the blood vessels of the vocal folds can become dilated and have an increased risk of rupturing, causing a hemorrhage into the fold. This can have devastating consequences on the voice. A good idea for a singer is to have allergy testing performed if allergies are suspected. This can allow for avoidance or modification of troublesome environments. If allergens are present, start with a topical steroid nasal spray as the first line of treatment. These can block allergic reactions with much less dying of the throat and larynx. If a topical steroid nasal spray (such as fluticasone in Flonase®) is not successful in controlling the symptoms, add an oral antihistamine on an as-needed basis. The oral agents are available at lower doses, and singers should always use the lowest dose possible to get the desired effect. Always try to have the antihistamine at the end of its dose interval at the time of a performance. For example, if using once-a-day loratadine (Claritin®), try to take the medication earlier in the day if you have an eveningperformance. By doing this, you will avoid singing while the medication reaches its peak levels in your body and the undesirable effects are greatest. Of all the over-the-counter antihistamines available, loratadine has the fewest side effects and should be considered the drug of choice for singers. If loratadine isn't strong enough, then try fexofenadine (Allegra®) or cetirizine (Zyrtec®). Cetirizine tends to be more sedating. A performer should always avoid any of the "D" formulas (such as Allegra® D or Zyrtec® D). The "D" stands for decongestant and most will have either 120 or 240 mg of pseudoephedrine. This is a very high dose and will be excessively drying and can even cause insomnia, hypertension, and rapid heart rates.

Commonly Used Over-the-Counter Antihistamines and Decongestants

azatadine (Trinalin®)

brompheniramine (Dimetane®)

cetirizine (Zyrtec®)

chlorpheniramine (Chlor-Trimeton®)

clemastine (Tavist®)
diphenhydramine (Benadryl®)
fexofenadine (Allegra®)
loratadine (Claritin®)
norepinephrine (Levophed®)
phenylephrine (Rynatan®)
pseudoephedrine (Sudafed®, Actifed®)

Prescription antihistamines

Prescription antihistamines are a newer generation of antihistamines that are less sedating than the over-the-counter brands. Despite the decreased likelihood of sedation, these medications can still cause fatigue or altered cognitive ability such as the sensation of being in a daze. As a class, these tend to be drying by both decreasing the amount of mucus produced and making the secretions thicker. Oral steroids, such as prednisone, are very effective at controlling allergy symptoms. A high dose of steroids used for just three days will eliminate the symptoms and will be less drying and sedating than using antihistamines. This is often the best treatment option to control an acute allergic reaction immediately before, or the day of, a performance. A longer-lasting steroid injection can also be very effective for controlling allergies for several weeks at a time.

Commonly Used Prescription Antihistamines
desloratadine (Clarinex®)
levocetirizine (Xyzal®)

Over-the-counter nasal sprays

Nasal sprays that are available over the counter are effective in decreasing nasal congestion and drainage. Sprays such as Afrin® (oxymetazoline) and Neo-Synephrine® can be safely used on a short-term basis. The time period should not exceed four to five days, because a rebound effect can occur that will increase the symptoms and the spray can become "addictive." Using a nasal spray for a cold or nasal congestion is better than using an oral drying agent such as pseudoephedrine. A nasal spray treats the problem more directly at the source with less systemic effects. It rapidly opens nasal passages and decreases drainage, lessening facial pressure and the feeling of congestion. It is a good choice for the treatment of a mild cold or to gain control of nasal symptoms due to allergies on the day of a performance.

Cromolyn (NasalCrom®) is the generic name for a nasal spray that was previously a prescription medication for the treatment of allergic rhinitis. This treatment is now out of date because the spray must be used four times a day to be effective and newer allergy sprays are more efficient. There are also other "natural" sprays that contain capsaicin[1] that appear safe and effective.

Saline nasal sprays used on a daily basis can improve the health of the nasal lining, keep nasal drainage thin, and even decrease the frequency of respiratory infections. To irrigate the nose with saline, you can choose from a few methods: a neti pot, a pressurized spray, or a squeeze bottle. You can also go online to see a slideshow demonstrating how to perform the irrigation: http://www.webmd.com/allergies/ss/slideshow-nasal-irrigation. The delivery methods are comparable and should be chosen based on your comfort and results. If you suffer from chronic sinus or rhinitis issues, this is a very healthy and safe addition to your daily routine.

Prescription nasal sprays

Steroid nasal sprays are an excellent way of treating allergy symptoms. These are more effective at controlling the symptoms than antihistamines. The sprays are very safe and are even approved for children down to the age of two. Nasal steroids work by blocking the reaction before it occurs instead of trying to block the reaction after it occurs like the antihistamines. The nasal steroid sprays are far less drying than the oral preparations. Sensitive individuals may develop throat irritation with these because some of the medication is swallowed. This irritation can be decreased by gently blowing the nose within a few minutes of using the spray. Another option is to use an antihistamine spray, which is very rapid in onset but can cause throat dryness and even mild sedation. All of these sprays are safe, and some are better tolerated than others. The best approach is to have a short trial period to decide on which spray works the best and is most tolerated by the individual.

Antihistamine Spray
solopatadine (Patanase®)
azelastine (Astelin®)

Intranasal Steroids
budesonide (Rhinocort®)
fluticasone (Flonase®, Veramyst®)
mometasone (Nasonex®)
triamcinolone (Nasacort®)

---

[1] Capsaicin is the phytochemical that makes some peppers, such as cayenne peppers, hot.

11.2 ANTIBIOTICS

Antibiotics are classified in many different families, such as penicillin, quinolones, sulfas, cephalosporins, and macrolides. The main active ingredient[2] determines their class. Antibiotics need to be used cautiously. In general, they can cause stomach upset and diarrhea. Antibiotics work by killing bacteria, both good and bad. Antibiotics weaken the body's normal flora and, as a result, a fungal overgrowth called *Candida albicans* or "thrush" can grow. This fungus can colonize the mouth, the throat, and even the larynx. Be sure to take an acidophilus (good bacteria) liquid or capsule-form supplement and eat foods that contain acidophilus (unsweetened yogurt and fermented soy products, such as miso and tempeh) while taking an antibiotic to help the body maintain its healthy flora.[3]

Antibiotics are only effective with *bacterial* infections (most upper respiratory infections are *viral*). As a general rule, they should be prescribed only when an upper respiratory infection has lasted seven to ten days. A throat culture should determine which antibiotic to prescribe. In general, the best antibiotics for sinus and respiratory infections are the quinolones, amoxicillin-clavulanate, and the macrolides. The stronger the antibiotic, the more likely it is to help you, but also the more likely the occurrence of side effects.

Penicillin
amoxicillin (Amoxil®)
amoxicillin-clavulanate (Augmentin®)—good for sinus and respiratory infections
ampicillin (Polycillin®)
penicillin (Pen V-K®)

Cephalosporins (related to penicillin, and a small percent of patients who are allergic to penicillin will be allergic to cephalosporins)
cefdinir (Omnicef®)
cefprozil (Cefzil®)
cefuroxime (Ceftin®)
cephalexin (Keflex®)

Macrolides (good for sinus and respiratory infections)
azithromycin (Zithromax®)
clarithromycin (Biaxin®)
erythromycin (Ery-Tab®)

---

[2] Also called the "base compound." Antibiotics are grouped according to whatever is in them that is killing or slowing the growth of bacteria.

[3] Acidophilus (Lactobacillus acidophilus)," last modified October 1, 2011,http://www.mayoclinic.com/health/lactobacillus/NS_patient-acidophilus, accessed July 1, 2012.

Quinolones (good for sinus and respiratory infections)
ciprofloxacin (Cipro®)
levofloxacin (Levaquin®)
moxifloxacin (Avelox®)

Tetracyclines
doxycycline (Doxy®)
tetracycline hydrochloride "Hcl" (Sumycin®)

Sulfonamides (Sulfa Drugs)
trimethoprim/sulfamethoxazole (Bactrim®)

11.3 ANXIETY MEDICATIONS/ANTIDEPRESSANTS/MOOD STABILIZERS

As a class, these medications tend to be very drying for the throat and vocal folds. They obviously alter mental capacity. These medications tend to cause sedation. These should be used with caution and only used after consulting with a physician. These medications tend to be overprescribed and dependency can develop. At the appropriate dose these medications can be very helpful and necessary for daily functioning. However, you need to determine if the benefits of the medication outweigh the potential side effects, or just accept the consequences and modify accordingly. All of the following medications have dryness and fatigue as side effects. Additional side effects are listed.

amitriptyline (Elavil®); loss of speech coordination, slurring
bupropion (Wellbutrin®)
citalopram (Celexa®); may trigger coughing, reflux, asthma, laryngitis, and bronchospasms
desipramine (Norpramin®); nausea
doxepin (Silenor®)
fluoxetine (Prozac®); sore throat, weakness, nausea
imipramine (Tofranil®)
nortriptyline (Pamelor®)
paroxetine (Paxil®); difficulty concentrating, lump in the throat, light sensitivity, runny nose, joint pain
protriptyline (Vivactil®); dizziness, black tongue, flushing
sertraline (Zoloft®); nervousness, sore throat, sweating
trazodone (Desyrel®)
trimipramine maleate (Surmontil®)
venlafaxine (Effexor®); weakness, headache, twitching, heartburn

Mental Disorder Medications/Antipsychotics

chlorpromazine (Thorazine®)

clozapine (Clozaril®)

fluphenazine (Permitil®, Prolixin®)

haloperidol (Haldol®)

loxapine (Loxitane®)

molindone (Moban®)

perphenazine (Trilafon®)

risperidone (Risperdal®); articulation difficulty

thioridazine (Mellaril®)

trifluoperazine (Stelazine®)

Anxiety Disorder Medications

benzodiazepine (all anxiety medications listed here fall under this classification);
  slurred speech (**dysarthria**)

alprazolam (Xanax®); loss of muscular coordination/nerve function; alters pitch,
  timbre, volume

chlordiazepoxide (Librax®)

clonazepam (Klonopin®)

diazepam (Valium®); weakness, nausea, blurred vision

lorazepam (Ativan®); tremor, weakness, dizziness, blurred vision

triazolam (Halcion®)

Central nervous system stimulants and attention deficit hyperactivity disorder medications

Attention deficit hyperactivity disorder (ADHD) has become a more recognized disorder in adults, and medical management with medication is becoming commonplace. This class of medication is associated with loss of fine muscle control/coordination, nervousness or restlessness, sleep disorders, and rapid heart rate.

dextroamphetamine (Adderall®)

methylphenidate (Ritalin®, Concerta®)

11.4 ASTHMA MEDICATIONS

Asthma and reactive airway diseases causing wheezing and allergic reactions can have a profound effect on the singing voice. The lungs provide the power source for driving the production of sound. When the air source is diminished, such as during an asthma flare-up, the length of time a singer can sing on one breath is reduced. With fluctuations in the amount of air, the vocal fold muscles need to frequently adjust the strength of their contraction to compensate and maintain the same volume. The breath support of the voice is decreased and vocal fatigue is more common. Consistent vocal performance can be compromised by poorly controlled asthma. In addition, the medications used to treat asthma can adversely affect the voice. Inhalers can result in vocal cord irritation, as they need to pass through the folds to reach the lungs. The more frequently the inhalers are needed, the more likely they are to produce irritation.

Asthma causes smooth muscle contraction in the small airways that decreases the amount of airflow in the lungs and produces a wheezing sound. Certain inhalers use a substance called a beta agonist to relax the muscles to open up the narrowed airways. Short-acting beta agonists, such as albuterol, are used as a "rescue" inhaler by asthmatics during attacks. Long-acting beta agonists, such as salmeterol, are used in combination with the steroid sprays. Long-acting beta agonists should never be used during an attack and are more of a maintenance medication. Both short- and long-acting forms can cause nervousness, tremor, rapid heart rate, and mucosa inflammation. Asthma is also associated with inflammation of the airways with increased mucus production, both of which are treated with steroid inhalers. The steroid inhalers can irritate the folds and cause swelling. The use of steroid inhalers also can lead to *Candida* infections (thrush) developing on the folds. This risk is decreased with the use of a "spacer" and by not using the dry powder forms of the inhaler (such as fluticasone propionate in the Advair Diskus®). Any inhaler can cause vocal fold dryness, leading to vocal fatigue and resulting in a raspy voice. This is more common with the heavier dry powder steroid inhalers. Singers with asthma should consider working with an asthma specialist (a pulmonologist or an allergist) with a goal of optimizing control with the lowest dose and frequency of inhalers. The addition of a leukotriene receptor antagonist, such as montelukast (Singulair®), that is delivered in pill form can control mild asthma or decrease the frequency and dose of inhaler use. Asthma and allergies are in a class of what is called atopic diseases, meaning that they can often occur together. Controlling the allergies will improve control of the asthma. Theophylline is an older form of treatment that is not commonly used. This medication can cause nervousness and dryness and the levels need to be monitored with blood tests to ensure appropriate dosing.

Short-Acting Beta Agonists
albuterol (Proventil®, Ventolin®, ProAir®, Combivent®)
metaproterenol (Alupent®)
pirbuterol (Maxair®)

Long-Acting Beta Agonists
formoterol (Foradil®, Symbicort®)
salmeterol (Serevent®, Advair®)

Steroid Inhalers
budesonide (Pulmicort®, Symbicort®)
beclomethasone (Beclovent®)

flunisolide (AeroBid®)
fluticasone (Advair®, Flovent®)
triamcinolone (Azmacort®)

Leukotriene Inhibitors
zileuton (Zyflo®)
montelukast (Singulair®)

11.5 BLOOD PRESSURE MEDICATIONS (ANTIHYPERTENSIVES)

Blood pressure control is very important to prevent complications such as a stroke or heart attack. There are many different classes of medications used to treat high blood pressure. The various classes each have different potential side effects.

Angiotensin-converting enzyme inhibitors (ACE Inhibitors)

This class of medication is used for blood pressure control and to treat congestive heart failure and to improve survival after heart attacks. One of the side effects of this class is to cause hoarseness due to laryngeal and throat swelling and a dry cough. This is reversible after stopping the medication. Other side effects include lightheadedness.

captopril (Capoten®)
enalapril (Vasotec®)
lisinopril (Prinivil®, Zestril®)
ramipril (Altace®)

Beta blockers

Beta blockers are also used to control heart rate and to protect the heart after a heart attack and are used in low doses to treat performance anxiety. These may dull vocal performance, flatten the affect, and/or cause dizziness and fatigue. These should not be used by patients with asthma.

atenolol (Tenormin®)
metoprolol (Lopressor®, Toprol®)
propranolol (Inderal®)

Calcium channel blockers

These are used to treat high blood pressure, control heart rate, and prevent chest pain. Side effects include lightheadedness, fatigue, and flu-like symptoms. This class can aggravate reflux and should be used with caution in singers with reflux disease.

amlodipine (Norvasc®)
nicardipine (Cardene®)
nifedipine (Procardia®)
verapamil (Calan®)
diltiazem (Cardizem®)

Diuretics

These are used to treat hypertension and fluid retention from kidney disease or heart failure. These work by taking fluid out of your body (diuresis) by producing more urine. Caffeine and alcohol are technically diuretics as well. By removing free fluid from the body, these medications can create dry mouth, muscle cramps, dizziness, and sore throat.

furosemide (Lasix®)
hydrochlorothiazide (Dyazide®, Maxzide®, Zestoretic®)—this is often used in combination with other blood pressure medications
spironolactone (Aldactone®)—deepening of the voice
triamterene (Dyrenium®)

11.6 BLOOD THINNERS

Blood thinners are used to decrease the chances of a clot forming in the body. They can be used on a short-term basis, such as with a blood clot in the legs, or on a long-term basis, such as with heart rhythm problems (atrial fibrillation). They are also used in patients with increased risk of heart attacks or strokes. Many over-the-counter medications used to treat pain, fevers, or arthritis also increase the risk of bleeding as a side effect. All of these medications need to be used with caution by singers. Singers with a history of a vocal cord hemorrhage should avoid these medications. The majority of these medications will increase the risk of bleeding for up to two weeks after taking the medication. Many of the "sinus" medications available over the counter contain blood thinners such as ibuprofen. Using medication to treat a "cold" prior to singing can be detrimental, as an upper respiratory infection causes the blood vessels around the vocal folds to become dilated (swollen), increasing the risk of bleeding with heavy use. Whenever a pain reliever is needed, acetaminophen (Tylenol®) should be used. It is *not* a blood thinner.

Strong Blood Thinners Used to Treat a Clot
warfarin (Coumadin®); given as a pill and requires regular blood testing to monitor levels

heparin (Lipo-Hepin®); given as intravenous medication

enoxaparin (Lovenox®); given as a shot

Platelet Aggregation Inhibitor

cilostazol (Pletal®)

clopidogrel (Plavix®)

prasugrel (Effient®)

Nonsteroidal Anti-Inflammatory Drugs (NSAIDs)

acetylsalicylic acid/aspirin (Bayer®, Bufferin®)

ibuprofen (Motrin®, Advil®)

naproxen (Aleve®)

11.7 COUGH SUPPRESSANTS (ANTITUSSIVES)

This group of medications decreases the urge to cough caused by tracheal secretions or swelling. Because these often contain codeine or a codeine derivative, they will cause sedation, fatigue, or imbalance as a side effect. The majority of cough suppressants are combined with mucus thinners such as guaifenesin. Despite the addition of a thinner, these medications will still cause dryness.

Commonly Used Cough Medications

benzonatate (Tessalon Perles®)

codeine (Tussi-Organidin®)

dextromethorphan (Robitussin® DM)

hydrocodone (Hycotuss®)

promethazine (Phenergan®)

11.8 DERMATOLOGIC DRUGS

A skin medication called isotretinoin (Accutane®, Amnesteem®, Claravis®, Sotret®) is a form of vitamin A that can be used to treat severe acne. This drug tends to produce a flushed feeling of the skin and increases the skin's sensitivity to sun exposure. It tends to cause system-wide dehydration, including the skin and throat, and can lead to voice changes such as decreased vocal agility, breathy tone, and loss of high notes. It has also been associated with depression and suicide, nausea, and blurred vision—all of which can have a detrimental effect on vocal performance. This powerful drug has other side effects not related to performance but serious enough to have made it illegal in several countries. Side effects tend to resolve soon after the patient stops taking the drug.

11.9 DIARRHEA MEDICATIONS/ANTISPASMODICS

Virtually all of these medications are very drying to the vocal folds and cause drowsiness and fatigue. Singers should use with caution.

diphenoxylate and atropine (Lomotil®)
loperamide (Imodium®)

11.10 GASTROINTESTINAL/REFLUX MEDICATIONS

Reflux is a very common cause of vocal difficulty. It is the most common noninfectious cause of hoarseness. It is important to realize that reflux cannot be cured, only controlled. It is also important to realize the refluxate, which is the fluid that leaves your stomach and enters the esophagus to reach the throat, has more in it than just acid. This fluid has enzymes, such as pepsin and bile, that also cause irritation. The irritation from reflux can be relieved with treatment, but once patients have a diagnosis of reflux they will always be prone to reflux in the future. The reflux can be controlled by behavioral modification if it is mild. More significant reflux requires daily or at least periodic medical treatment. If a singer has been diagnosed with reflux causing vocal swelling or irritation, medical treatment is needed. Once the swelling and irritation have occurred, relying on dietary and behavioral modifications to resolve the damage and recurrences requires an extended period of time. Taking a reflux medication will work quickly and efficiently to prevent a repeat reflux episode and avoid the exacerbation of or return of symptoms. There are several options available for the medical treatment of reflux. The most effective medication is a class known as proton pump inhibitors (PPIs). This class can be a prescription or over the counter. If you are treating only occasional indigestion or heartburn, then over-the-counter medications are sufficient. If you are experiencing reflux symptoms more than once a week, seek medical attention and consider reflux maintenance therapy in order to prevent any damage. Once the vocal fold irritation has resolved, it is important to treat any reflux symptoms that occur. This may be as simple as using antacids to neutralize the irritation. Be proactive in taking preventative measures. If eating certain foods or drinking alcohol causes reflux symptoms, then pretreat with an H_2 blocker or possibly a proton pump inhibitor to prevent the events from taking place.

Antacids

Antacids neutralize stomach acid and provide rapid relief of symptoms. The primary deficiency of this class of medication is that the control they provide is temporary. These are very short acting and are not a good choice for maintaining reflux in the long run. These have been combined with other longer-acting medications to get the benefit of both (e.g., Pepcid® Complete and Zegerid®). All of these have few side effects but can cause stomach upset, constipation, or dry mouth.

calcium carbonate (Tums®)

sodium bicarbonate (Alka-Seltzer®)—this is a combination with acetylsalicylic acid, which can increase the risk of bleeding

H_2 Blockers

H_2 blockers are an older class of medications that were previously prescription brand names only. These are now all available in generic and over-the-counter forms. They have very few side effects but can cause abdominal cramping and diarrhea.

cimetidine (Tagamet®)
famotidine (Pepcid®)
nizatidine (Axid®)
ranitidine (Zantac®)

Proton pump inhibitor

This class is the best at decreasing the amount of acid in the stomach. Most of these are available now as a generic or over-the-counter form. These can cause stomach pain, constipation, muscle cramps, and dry mouth. Long term use may harm bone health.

omeprazole (Prilosec®, Zegerid®)
esomeprazole (Nexium®)
lansoprazole (Prevacid®)
rabeprazole (AcipHex®)
pantoprazole (Protonix®)

11.11 HORMONE THERAPY

Birth control pills can lead to vocal cord swelling and changes to the voice. Females need to pay close attention and listen for any changes after starting the medication. Voice changes from "the pill" will cease when the medication is no longer taken. Progesterone, which is part of the birth control pill, can cause fluid retention affecting range and voice quality. Other hormones, such as danazol (Danocrine®), used for endometriosis and fibrocystic breast disease can cause deepening of the voice that can be permanent.

11.12 NAUSEA/MOTION SICKNESS/ANTIDIZZINESS MEDICATIONS

These medications are associated with significant dry mouth, blurred vision, and sedative effects.

dimenhydrinate (Dramamine®)

meclizine (Antivert®)

prochlorperazine (Compazine®)

promethazine (Phenergan®)

ondansetron (Zofran®)—newer form of antinausea medication. This is commonly
   used after surgery and during chemotherapy.

scopolamine (Transderm Scop®)

11.13 MUCOLYTICS

Mucus-thinning agents can be used to counteract the drying effects of other medications. Mucolytics are not a substitute for adequate hydration. These are beneficial when performing in very dry climates. Another instance of dehydration occurs from airplane travel. The dry and low-humidity air in the plane's pressurized cabin will cause water loss from the body. As a general rule, at least eight ounces of water is required for each hour of travel. Mucolytics are relatively harmless and are beneficial for most performers under the appropriate conditions. The primary drug in mucolytics is guaifenesin. This was once a prescription commonly used by singers called Humibid® LA, but it is now available over the counter as Mucinex®. Mucinex® is a must for performers to have available when traveling. Mucolytics have minimal side effects and can be taken as often as necessary; however, they work best if you don't use them every day. Guaifenesin stimulates the water component of serous mucus and works best if you are well hydrated. Be sure to take it with water. Guaifenesin doesn't produce more saliva; it just thins out what you have available. It is not a substitute for poor water intake. The body will adjust and return to what it was doing before in people whose saliva is naturally tacky.

There are cases of more severe dryness that may not respond to mucolytics. Severe dryness can be medication induced, or it can also be due to Sjögren's syndrome, a primary autoimmune disorder or a secondary disorder (developing later in life) associated with rheumatoid arthritis. Sjögren's syndrome usually causes severe dryness of the mouth (xerostomia), laryngeal dryness (laryngeal sicca), hoarseness, and a burning sensation that is aggravated by singing. This condition requires more aggressive treatment with pilocarpine (Salagen®) or cevimeline (Evoxac®). These medications can be used daily for severe cases or as needed for laryngeal dryness that does not respond to guaifenesin. (See 10.18 Laryngeal Sicca.)

11.14 PAIN RELIEVERS

Narcotics

Narcotics are controlled substances and only available (legally) by prescription. These all are associated with dry throat, sedation, lethargy, decreased reaction time, and flat affect. Nausea is a common side effect. These can also result in slurred speech (dysarthria) and uninhibited or diminished compulsion to speak.

acetaminophen and codeine (Tylenol® #3)
acetaminophen and hydrocodone (Vicodin®, Lortab®)
acetaminophen and oxycodone (Endocet®, Percocet®)
acetaminophen and propoxyphene (Propacet®, Darvocet®)

Nonsteroidal anti-inflammatory drugs (NSAIDs)

These pain relievers need to be used with caution when performing because they decrease the sensation of the larynx and may mask a potential problem. They will affect mental ability and can result in slurred speech. Try to avoid the many pain relievers that are also anti-inflammatory medications or aspirin-containing products. These are often suggested for laryngeal pain or irritation, but because they thin the blood, they will increase the risk of a vocal fold hemorrhage. Use headache, sinus, and cold preparations with caution as aspirin is often added to these for pain relief. When a pain reliever is absolutely necessary, a singer's safest choice is to use acetaminophen (Tylenol®) because it is not a blood thinner and, of all the pain killers, it has the fewest side effects.

Over-the-Counter Examples
acetaminophen (Tylenol®)
acetylsalicylic acid/aspirin (Bayer®, Bufferin®)
ibuprofen (Advil®, Motrin®, Nuprin®)
naproxen (Aleve®, Naprosyn®)

Prescription Examples
celecoxib (Celebrex®); This is what is called a cyclooxygenase-2 (COX-2) inhibitor
    and it is commonly used for the treatment of arthritic conditions. Unlike the
    other NSAIDs, celecoxib is not associated with increased bleeding.
nabumetone (Relafen®); dry mouth, mouth sores, dizziness
oxaprozin (Daypro®); dizziness and drowsiness
piroxicam (Feldene®); can cause hoarseness and dizziness

11.15 SLEEP AIDS

Sleep aids need to be used with caution. This class of medication can be addictive if used over time. The side effects include dryness and altered mental status that can carry over into the daytime. Sleep aids can also decrease muscle coordination and physical performance. Short-term use can be safe. For instance, if you need help with insomnia while traveling, consider a short-acting medication to minimize daytime mental capability. There are many different types of sleeping aids.

Herbal Medications: melatonin

Antihistamines: diphenhydramine (Benadryl®)

Antidepressants: amitriptyline (Elavil®)

Hypnotics: eszopiclone (Lunesta®); zolpidem (Ambien®)

11.16 STEROIDS

Corticosteroids are very different from the anabolic steroids some bodybuilders use illegally. Anabolic steroids, whether taken orally, injected, or via skin patch, increase muscle mass and result in the permanent masculinization of the voice. Corticosteroids, on the other hand, are anti-inflammatory and are miracle drugs when used in the right setting. They combat the vocal changes associated with swelling from overuse, with swelling due to vocal fold nodules or polyps, and most commonly with upper respiratory infections with associated laryngitis. The effects can be dramatic and can save a performance.

Corticosteroids, such as prednisone, have been used for decades. They are the quickest and strongest way to treat allergic reactions and are most commonly used to treat patients with severe asthma. They are used to decrease swelling and open the airway during an exacerbation of an asthma attack. Long-acting corticosteroid shots are used to treat environmental allergies and poison ivy (the latter of which can also be treated with topical corticosteroids). Corticosteroids are given orally in pill form or as a shot in the muscle or vein to treat vocal fold swelling due to any cause. The method depends on the time available before the need to use the voice. If a performer has at least six hours before requiring voice, then an oral application should be used. When only a few hours are available, intramuscular (IM) injection is more efficient. Only in rare cases when less than an hour is available is an intravenous (IV) injection used.

All steroids are not the same. The anti-inflammatory properties are different, and patients respond differently to the different preparations. Dexamethasone (Decadron®) has superior anti-inflammatory properties over prednisone, for instance. Steroids can have adverse side effects. Short-term effects include irritability, agitation, and insomnia. Appetite increases while on steroids as well. Diabetics need to use steroids with caution as the blood sugar levels increase while taking the medication. Long-term effects include abnormal fat deposits leading to a rounding of the face ("moon face") and a hump formation on the back, as well as a loss of bone density (osteoporosis). Usually these effects only occur with continuous steroid use over months. Avascular necrosis of the femoral head (loss of a portion of the hip bone) can occur with either short- or long-term steroid use. Most singers report that the vocal folds do not feel normal while on steroids but have a heavy feeling.

Steroids can be used safely when used for the appropriate reasons and setting. They can allow a singer to complete a performance that otherwise would not have been possible. The importance of the performance needs to be considered. Vocal professionals need to make prudent use of steroids and minimize the duration of their use. Steroid use should be limited to one week or less whenever possible. Steroids do not make the voice invincible, and they do not eliminate the need to rest the voice. Rather, they allow a performer to postpone voice rest to get through a performance. Once the course of steroids is complete, voice rest should be taken, potentially followed by voice therapy. Voice professionals must carefully follow the regimen their physician prescribes to lessen the risk of a detrimental rebound effect on the voice following the steroids. If steroids are required more than once a year, the physician and patient need to determine the underlying problem. If used consistently more than once a year, adverse side effects can occur. Steroids are not addictive, but singers can become dependent on them to get through performances. Singers with a vocal fold pathology, such as a polyp, can become dependent on steroids to decrease not only the swelling that accompanies their pathology but also the additional swelling that develops from singing with the pathology. Without the steroids they cannot sing or cannot sing for more than a short period of time. The pathology needs to be addressed instead of masking the effects with potentially dangerous medication. Touring performers can abuse the medication as they may obtain the steroids from several different physicians or other performers while on the road.

Corticosteroids
dexamethasone (Decadron®)
methylprednisolone (Medrol® Dosepak)
hydrocortisone (Hydrocortone®, Solu-Cortef®)
prednisone (Deltasone®)

11.17 HERBAL MEDICATIONS

Herbal medications, such as traditional Chinese medication, have been used for centuries with success. These are not subject to Food and Drug Administration (FDA) approval and can be associated with numerous side effects. We mention a few for their potential to cause vocal edema due to hormonal shifts and some others for putting the vocal folds at risk for hemorrhaging, but all herbal medicines should be used with caution.[4]

(See Singing on Swollen Vocal Folds in 3.9 Vocal Hazards.)

- Dong quai "female ginseng" increases ovarian and testicular hormonal production.
- Yam has progesterone-like properties.

---

[4] For a more extensive and descriptive list of herbal effects, log on to http://www.herbmed.org. For more information about herbal supplements and medications, log on to MedicineNet.com: http://www.focusonmedications.com/script/main/hp.asp.

- Licorice root causes estrogen- and progesterone-type effects and can raise blood pressure.
- Primrose enhances estrogen production.
- Melatonin assists estrogen and progesterone production.
- Yohimbe may enhance testosterone production.
- Feverfew, garlic, ginger, gingko biloba, Saint John's wort, and ginseng can interfere with blood clotting or dilate blood vessels and thin the blood, lowering the threshold for vocal fold hemorrhaging.

Anecdotes to emphasize the effectiveness of herbs:

1. As a tired new mom, I (Dr. Rachael Gates) enjoyed a tea that advertised a calming effect. I found it relaxed me to have a cup each evening before bed and helped me get to sleep. After a couple weeks, I began experiencing dizziness episodes and unusual fatigue. At first I attributed these to being sleep deprived, but I visited the doctor to be certain. The doctor checked my vitals and discovered that I had low blood pressure. Both of us were confused by the low numbers, but my symptoms seemed to agree with the finding. That evening, I looked up the first ingredient in the calming tea online (passionflower) and found that it causes low blood pressure!

2. Licorice root is delicious and is found in some black licorice and added to many herbal teas for a sweet aftertaste. It can raise blood pressure considerably, however, and can even cause voice changes. My husband, a thirty-five-year-old who, at 6 feet 4 inches and 180 lbs, is physically very fit, was enjoying one cup of licorice root tea every evening for a couple of weeks while preparing for an ultramarathon. He checked his vital statistics and was shocked to discover his blood pressure was quite high. The tea was the culprit. His blood pressure returned to normal within a week after he stopped drinking the tea. The moral? Enjoy the benefits and yummy tastes herbs can offer, but respect their potency.

11.18 VITAMIN SUPPLEMENTS

Some vitamin supplements have the potential to alter your voice or put you at higher risk for a vocal pathology. Below are a few commonly taken supplements that should be used with caution.

- Niacin and vitamin E can dilate blood vessels and thin the blood, lowering the threshold for vocal fold hemorrhaging.
- Vitamin C is a diuretic and can be very drying if consumed in large doses.[5] (See High Doses of Vitamin C in 3.9 Vocal Hazards.)

---

[5] Anthony Jahn, "Vitamins and Herbal Medicines: All Good?" *Classical Singer,* December 2001, 22.

12

Cautions to the Singer Undergoing Surgery

12.1 ASPECTS OF THE SURGICAL PROCESS THAT CONCERN SINGERS

REGARDLESS OF TYPE, any surgery performed on a singer presents unique concerns demanding special consideration from all those involved. Because most physicians are not professional singers, and because their primary aim is to keep you alive at all costs, voice preservation is not top priority. Do not assume just because you tell them you are a professional singer that they will understand how to protect your instrument during the surgical process. As a general rule, you should be very conservative when dealing with any surgery. Always weigh the risks involved with the benefits of any surgery. You can avoid many complications by observing the following precautions.

Back-to-back scheduling

It is commonly known that more surgical errors (including anesthesiology, nursing care, etc.) occur later in the day when surgical teams are tired. When selecting a date for your surgery, consider asking how many surgeries are scheduled around you and request as early a time as possible. Having a surgery earlier in the day also means that plenty of staff will still be on duty to assist if you have problems after surgery such as nausea and vomiting.

General anesthesia

General anesthesia involves the administering of strong muscle relaxants that are so effective that you appear asleep. Your entire body relaxes, including your stomach, making it much more difficult to hold down food. The placement of the endotracheal tube before surgery and its removal after surgery will make you susceptible to gagging and throwing up anything in the stomach. Throwing up is very important to avoid after a vocal fold operation, because the strain and acidic regurgitation can irritate the freshly cut vocal folds. Additionally, throwing up when you're in a groggy state puts you at a high risk of aspirating (inhaling) the vomit into the lungs and getting pneumonia or even choking and dying. The risk is greatest as you're going to sleep. To help decrease your risk of aspirating, you must refrain from eating and drinking for eight hours prior to surgery. The absorption of anesthesia into your body's tissues is optimized by an empty stomach as well. You are permitted to sip some clear liquids, however, such as water, weak herbal tea (with or without sugar), and diluted apple juice up to four hours prior to surgery because they pass through the stomach quickly and easily. Be sure to keep these to a minimum, however, to avoid any chance of your surgery being cancelled.

Note: Although Sprite® is a clear liquid, it's not recommended because its carbonation aggravates reflux.

Note: A man who drank orange juice the morning of his surgery had to be rescheduled for his operation.

Anesthetics are absorbed by the body's fatty tissues, and the quickest way to shed their aftereffects, such as nausea, drowsiness, and minor coordination problems, is by getting up and moving. Movement and sweat help break up and flush the body of stored anesthetic remnants. Because vocal folds don't contain fatty tissue, they do not need such exercise right away. In fact, because general anesthesia weakens the body's energy levels, a period of voice rest is recommended. Any nonlaryngeal surgery requiring general anesthesia should be followed with one to two days of complete voice rest, no singing for the first week, and no performing for the first two weeks. On the other hand, phonosurgeries and other laryngeal surgeries requiring general anesthesia will follow with longer periods of voice rest and more restrictions. (See 12.1 Aspects of the Surgical Process That Concern Singers and Voice Rest in 12.2 Postoperation Concerns.)

Intubation

Intubation is the insertion of an endotracheal tube used to ventilate the lungs of a patient under general anesthesia. The intubation process poses many threats to singers. If a surgeon decides a procedure on a singer mandates the administration of general anesthesia, his **anesthesiologist** performing the intubation should be very well trained and highly experienced. Damage from the tube's insertion can be worse than what you're trying to repair. Because the folds will automatically spasm shut when anything touches close to them (see 2.4 The Many Functions of the Larynx), the anesthesiologist must first put the patient to sleep and then add a strong muscle relaxant to the patient's intravenous (IV) drip to help relax the folds.

Note: If a muscle relaxant is added to the intravenous drip before the patient reaches an unconscious or "asleep" state, the patient will be unable to breathe but will still be awake. This is called intraoperative awareness and is very frightening for a patient.

He should then generously spray lidocaine on the folds to numb them and decrease their ability to perceive the interference. (Request the lidocaine spray! Most anesthesiologists don't know to do this!) Damage can be done to the folds as the endotracheal tube is inserted prior to surgery or removed following surgery. The risk of damage is greater if the patient's folds are not completely paralyzed and try to shut as the tube passes through. Damage such as bruising or arytenoid dislocation may occur if the glottis is narrow from incomplete abduction, or if the patient's anatomy prohibits a good view (e.g., a short neck and fat tongue combination), but especially if the anesthesiologist is inexperienced or rough. The left vocal fold is more frequently injured in the placement of the tube, because anesthesiologists are taught to hold the endoscope in their left hand in order to view what they are doing and actually place the endotracheal tube with the right hand. This causes the endotracheal tube to go in at a slight angle aimed more toward the left fold. Granuloma, scarring, or even paralysis of the vocal fold can result from the prolonged use of an endotracheal tube. The tube may irritate the epithelial layer of the vocal folds, resulting in soreness and hoarseness postsurgery. You may involuntarily gag, throw up, shake your head and neck, or cough in attempt to expel the obstruction while it's being removed, and as a result, your vocal folds may grind against the tube, irritating the folds. Because of this possibility, anyone having phonosurgery should be given antinausea medication in their IV fluid prior to the surgery. Other potential injuries include the endotracheal tube—or even the metal intubating laryngoscope—cutting the tongue, soft palate, or throat lining.

Any time a laser is used to operate on the upper airway (i.e., the tonsils, tongue, vocal folds, etc.), a special endotracheal tube is required for intubation. A regular plastic endotracheal tube lying between the vocal folds can catch fire when in proximity to the laser's heat. The fire would easily burn through the plastic tube, combine with the oxygen inside the tube, and cause a deadly explosion in the larynx. Instead, a tube coated with fire-resistant material is used. Unfortunately, the tube is often ribbed with metal and tends to irritate the folds as it rests between them. (See Figures 10.6b, 15.3a, and 15.3c.)

One of the more common complications associated with the intubation process is damage to the teeth. The metal laryngoscope sometimes used for oral intubation (as well as the metal operating laryngoscope used to perform microlaryngeal surgery) can chip, break, or even completely knock out a tooth. Loss of a tooth or teeth substantially hinders articulation in speaking and singing. The size of the scope is often the culprit. Using smaller-sized scopes will minimize the likelihood of damage.

Before the endotracheal tube is placed, the neck is propped up with a cushion and the head suspended back, naturally opening the jaw. A rigid metal half-cylinder scope with a light source on the end is inserted into the mouth along the blade of the tongue and positioned either under or over the epiglottis. The scope behaves much like a shoe horn, elevating the jaw and tongue and exposing a clear view of the glottis. Following the center of the tongue, the endotracheal tube is then inserted straight in until it rests between the vocal folds and in the upper third of the trachea. (See Figure 12.1a.)

When available, an intubating video laryngoscope (such as a Storz® or GlideScope® Video Laryngoscope) is preferable to the traditional rigid metal intubating scope in assisting with the placement of the tube. A videoscope has a camera on a specially shaped scope that inserts quickly and easily with the patient's head in a natural position. The camera on the inserted videoscope offers a clear view of the vocal folds, which it projects onto a screen, helping to safely guide endotracheal tube placement. Once the endotracheal tube is placed, the metal laryngoscope or videoscope—whichever is being used—is removed. The tube is then taped to the side of your mouth closest to the anesthesiologist, so as to make room for the insertion of the operating laryngoscope to be fitted centrally.

Due to the dangers intubation poses for the vocal folds, alternative methods have been developed but unfortunately are not often employed. One such option is the laryngeal mask airway (LMA). (See Figure 12.1b.) Developed by a British anesthetist in the

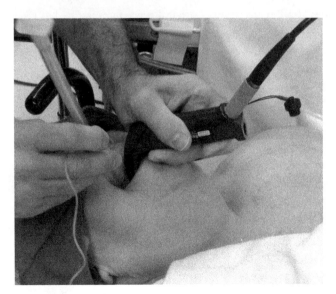

FIGURE 12.1a Intubation
Intubating a patient using a GlideScope®. The video laryngoscope is shown here being held in the left hand and the endotracheal tube is being inserted with the right.

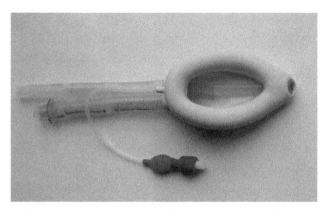

Figure 12.1b Laryngeal Mask Airway
Shown here with the cuff inflated.

mid-1980s, the LMA is a cuffed cup that rests along the base of tongue, over top of the epiglottis, and **aryepiglottic folds**. Once in place, the cuff surrounding the cup is inflated, sealing off the airway from above the vocal folds. An oxygen tube is passed through the mouth and attached to the cup, effectively ventilating the lungs without any disturbance to the vocal folds or trachea. At the very worst, the LMA will cause mild pharyngeal edema and erythema. This makes it an ideal choice, especially for emergency ventilating when vocal fold damage is often done with hurried intubations. Unfortunately, because the mask fits over the base of the tongue, it prevents access to the larynx and cannot be used for voice surgeries or other procedures involving the upper aerodigestive tract. Its use is also limited to short surgical procedures lasting less than one hour during which muscle relaxation is not needed (e.g., bladder, arm, leg, or foot surgeries).[1] Whenever possible, the LMA should replace endotracheal tube intubation in professional voice users.

Appropriate Tube Size

It is easier and faster to ventilate your lungs with air using a larger tube than a smaller one. In most cases, the anesthesiologist will want to intubate using the largest tube you can possibly tolerate (usually an 8 mm or 9 mm) unless the surgeon specifically requests a smaller size. Using a larger than necessary tube to intubate, however, can cause many vocal complications and should be avoided. Although many conscientious laryngologists visit

---

[1] Anesthesiologist, Kenneth Paul Gross, MD, of Associated Anesthesiologists, Lincoln, NE, e-mail message to author, January 7, 2011.

anesthesiology departments to educate on the vocal complications of using larger endotracheal tubes, little is done to enforce using smaller tubes. Ask your laryngologist what the smallest endotracheal tube size would be for your trachea. Sizes run from 1 mm (#1.0) for tiny babies to 10 mm (#10.0) for very large men. Anesthesiologists will generally opt for a #8.0 or #9.0 to service most adults. However, depending on your individual anatomical framework, adult males can usually tolerate a #7.0 and adult females a #6.0. Under almost any condition, these tube sizes are adequate to ventilate. There is a 20% chance the recurrent laryngeal nerve (RLN) will be damaged when an endotracheal tube larger than #7.5 is inserted in a man and #7.0 is inserted in a woman.[2] Insist that the anesthesiologist performing your intubation be someone well acquainted with the risk to singers' vocal folds. Ask your surgeon if there is a certain anesthesiologist with whom he prefers working. Request to meet the anesthesiologist prior to your surgery. Ask that he take his time and use the smallest tube possible—preferably the size recommended by the laryngologist.

> Note: If you're having vocal fold surgery, a smaller endotracheal tube allows better visibility of and accessibility to the vocal folds.
>
> Anesthesiologist, Dr. Kenneth P. Gross, e-mail message to author, January 7, 2011.

> Note: Keep your recommended endotracheal tube size in all your physicians' files as an emergency precaution.

Laser use

The use of a laser on vocal folds should be done with extreme caution, because it's never certain what the intense heat will do to surrounding tissues (e.g., possible **thermal damage**). Lasers should be used at the lowest power needed and only for very brief (0.05-second) impulse durations with time between pulses to allow the laser to cool and minimize lateral thermal injury.

> Note: Currently, the KTP (potassium titanyl phosphate) laser is the laser of choice for singers. The KTP is a green light beam set at a low power for photocoagulation. The laser plume or smoke while using the KTP is minimal as this laser uses almost no heat and causes the least thermal damage of the lasers.

---

[2] P. M. Santos, A. Afrassiabi, and E. A. Weymuller Jr., "Risk Factors Associated With Prolonged Intubation and Laryngeal Injury," *Otolaryngology Head and Neck Surgery* 111, no. 4 (October 1994): 453.

Schedule around menstruation

When scheduling any surgery, women should be operated upon within the first two weeks after their periods. Four to five days prior to menstruation, tissues are swollen and, as a result, less tolerant to absorbing anesthesia. Bloating can also interfere with structural definition, making anatomical structures less distinct. Patients undergoing surgery any later in their cycle increase the likelihood of adverse reactions to the anesthesia, such as nausea. Throwing up after phonosurgery is particularly undesirable due to the stress placed on freshly cut tissue and possible acid spillage on vulnerable laryngeal wounds.

Ingested interference

Although little blood is lost when operating on vocal folds, vocal fold surgery candidates are asked not to ingest any aspirin or other anticoagulants (Motrin®, Advil®, Aleve®, Excedrin®, Bayer®, Alka-Seltzer®, Anacin®, Bufferin®) for two weeks prior to surgery. This helps avoid unnecessary bleeding and hemorrhaging. Many herbal teas and supplements and even some vitamin supplements can interfere and should be stopped temporarily as well. (See Chapter 11, Vocally Hazardous Drugs.) Tobacco, alcohol, caffeine, and some over-the-counter and prescription medications (e.g., diet pills and other stimulants that affect heart rate) can affect the absorption and tolerance of general anesthesia. Be sure to give a list of every supplement, medication, and herbal tea you are consuming to the physician and anesthesiologist before scheduling the operation so that you can prepare accordingly. You may take approved, noninterfering oral medications (such as Tylenol®) with one ounce of water up to one hour before surgery. You will be allowed to resume taking other medications after the surgery is complete, so be sure to bring any prescriptions with you on the day of surgery. If you are on reflux medication, for example, resume taking it the day of surgery.

Scarring

Once wounded, the body heals itself by forming a stronger, less flexible fibrous tissue in the wound's place known as a scar. Scars that form along the soft palate or **tonsillar pillars** can inhibit the soft palate's ability to raise, not only limiting range, but also affecting resonance. If formed anywhere in or along the vocal folds, the scar's lack of elasticity may limit vocal fold vibration and range.

The key to beautiful phonation lies in preserving the vocal folds' layered structure, and the layers that make up the cover must be maintained at all costs. These wet layers become very slippery and elastic when well hydrated. They allow the two folds to easily slip against each other in smooth wave-like motions during phonation while simultaneously sliding around each other inside each fold as well. Hydrated cover layers minimize friction and soften the impact of each vibration so that you can speak and sing for long periods of time with ease. Because they are the folds' outermost layers, they are the most vulnerable to damage and need to be treated the most delicately during an operation. Even a minor scar in the raw egg white–like epithelium can become a dry spot on the tissue that can no longer retain moisture or vibrate well. When surgery is an absolute necessity, the surgeon should cut laterally to the free portion of the fold and lift and work underneath the cover whenever possible. By doing so, the cover can be relaid with as little disruption as possible and the medial edge remains smooth and uncut. (See Intubation and Appropriate Tube Size in 12.1 Aspects of the Surgical Process that Concern Singers.)

The folds' edges must be completely smooth and flexible to vibrate well and produce a clean, clear sound. They must be elastic to elongate for higher pitches. They must be smooth and wet to be able to seal together and prevent air from leaking through every time the folds come together during a vibration. Whenever surgery is concerned, the edges are at risk due to possible intubation trauma but especially when operated on directly. Stiff tissue that forms along the vibrating edge may prohibit the folds from completely closing when adducted, resulting in a breathy and hoarse vocal quality. Maintaining clean medial edge closure must be of primary importance to the surgeon operating on the vocal folds. Vocal fold surgery should be performed so that the least amount of tissue is removed to preserve closure for clean phonation. If too much vocal fold tissue is removed, a gap will remain and air will leak during phonation, resulting in a breathy, poor-quality sound.

After any surgery, rehabilitation therapy must begin as soon as the appropriate rest time is complete to prevent stiffening during healing. Beginning rehabilitation immediately following voice rest is especially important for vocal fold surgeries, after which the folds must be carefully and consistently stretched to loosen scar tissue as it forms. (See Voice Rest in 12.2 Postoperation Concerns.)

As we age, our body's responses slow and take longer to heal. During our teenage years and early twenties, however, the body is designed to go above and beyond the call of duty to heal itself. The body exuberantly heals skin incisions during this period of life when we are most likely to take careless risks and act impulsively by scarring easily, quickly, and abundantly (hypertrophic scar formation). You can help avoid overly abundant scarring by postponing surgeries when possible until after thirty years of age.

Note: This period of hypertrophic scar formation occurs only in skin/epidermis and does not affect vocal fold epithelium.

Skeletal structure

Maintaining the skeletal structure must be fundamental to surgeons operating on singers. Because singers use their entire bodies to sing, skeletal alignment must be intact to sing freely and efficiently. Great care must be taken to ensure that all anatomical scaffolding be protected. The hyoid bone, which may seem to take little part in phonation, functions to keep the airway open and to stabilize the larynx for singing. Even the scarring that forms after a bone is broken may inhibit singing, especially if the bone is a rib bone. Beware of any surgeries involving the chest, back, neck, or cervical spine as these can lead to the damage of cartilages and bones that inhibit singing and/or the vocal mechanism.

Muscular network

Because skeletal alignment must be intact to sing, so too must muscles be preserved to not only support the skeleton and the erect posture essential to singing but also support the respiration and the vocal mechanism. Generally, after initial surgical incisions through skin and fat layers, muscle is not actually cut, but separated. Beware of surgeries requiring the cutting or separating of abdominal muscles, such as cesarean sections, hysterectomies, and appendectomies. Abdominal muscle rehabilitation is necessary following such surgeries in order to regain strength to support singing. Head and neck surgeries, such as cervical nodule removal and thyroid surgery, also often involve the separation of muscles in the neck that attach to the hyoid bone and stabilize the larynx. Such surgeries can scar in a way that inhibits vertical laryngeal movement and laryngeal stability necessary for swallowing and phonation. Facial muscles must be carefully preserved as well for emoting, diction, and resonance.

Note: The larynx can travel vertically about 7 cm. If you put a finger on the front of your neck and swallow and yawn, you can feel this range of motion.

Nerve damage

The superior laryngeal nerve (SLN) and RLN must not be harmed. Due to their routes, the SLN and RLN are susceptible to damage during surgeries (or chest or neck injuries). The surgeon should have an excellent understanding of the location of the nerves and take care not to place them in harm's way. A pinch, a nick from a knife, or even just the pressure of a retracting tool moving one of these nerves aside can irreparably alter their ability to control vocal range, pitch, and loudness. The nerves do have the ability to repair themselves, but there is a chance they may not recover depending on the severity of the injury. These nerves are at the highest risk (up to 10% of the time) during thyroid, parathyroid, and cervical herniated disc surgeries but are also commonly damaged in patients having vascular neck, chest, heart, lung, carotid artery (**endarterectomy**), cystic hygroma, thyroglossal duct cyst, and bronchial cyst surgery.

Facial nerves must also be preserved for emoting, diction, and resonance. Facial nerve injuries result in facial paralysis and can occur from procedures on the ear, mastoid, or salivary gland.

Respiratory weakening

Air production and respiratory function efficiency must be preserved to maintain sub-glottal pressure and vocal fold vibration. Ribcage and chest wall surgeries interfere with respiratory function and must be followed with pulmonary function rehabilitation to avoid chest wall stiffening in the healing process. Abdominal surgery hinders respiratory support as well. To enter the abdominal cavity, abdominal muscles must be cut that help produce and maintain the subglottal pressure needed to phonate, as well as execute octave leaps and **coloratura** (agility). Among other surgeries, open **laparotomies** inflict much postoperative pain and mandate long recoveries of six to twelve weeks. Under such conditions, normal vocal practice regimens are virtually impossible and should be avoided until the singer has fully recovered in order to prevent developing poor habits that compensate for the lack of breath support.

Resonator alteration

Any operation performed in the oral, pharyngeal, or nasal cavity may alter resonance and, in turn, change the sound of the voice. Common surgeries, such as facelifts, sinus surgeries, tonsillectomies, dental extractions, nasal septoplasties, adenoidectomies, and turbinate reductions, can change vocal resonance. These vocal changes are not always desirable and may not only disrupt a singer's trademark sound but also make achieving a desirable sound more difficult. Occasionally surgeries that alter resonator cavities will improve the sound of the voice. Removing large tonsils or severe nasal blockage due to sinus inflammation or a **deviated nasal septum** will allow more air and vibrations to reach the resonating cavities and may improve the singer's voice quality, as well as his or her awareness of desirable resonance vibrations. Surgery that changes resonance should be carefully considered because a positive vocal outcome cannot be ensured and will most certainly demand relearning, to some degree, vocal technique and new sensations felt during phonation.

Articulator alteration

A singer's tongue, teeth, hard palate, soft palate, jaw, lips, and glottis must be protected and remain fully functional for beautiful singing. Mouthguards are usually in place throughout microlaryngeal surgery to protect the teeth from the metal scope and surgical instruments inserted into the mouth. (See Figure 12.5a.) Beware of tongue surgery, temporomandibular joint surgery, and orthodontic procedures. Tonsils should only be removed when absolutely necessary, because a tonsillectomy can scar your soft palate to the point of tethering the tissue. (See Tonsillitis in 12.3 Common Problems Where Surgery Could Affect the Vocal Mechanism.) If your soft palate becomes tethered from scarring, it will have a limited ability to elevate and may be unable to reach the back of the throat to close off the nasal passageway for talking and singing. Air will then leak into the nose during speaking and singing, making the voice hypernasal. In this case, palatal strengthening exercises are an important part of the recovery process, and some minor changes in singing technique may be required to help close the velum to the back of the throat. The soft palate could, on the other hand, scar overabundantly, blocking the passageway to the nose so that words like "mom" and "note" come out hyponasally as "bob" and "dote."

Many singers, however, will notice an improvement in the resonating cavity when very large tonsils or nasal blockages are successfully removed with minimal scarring. Their removal opens up the resonating cavity, often improving the quality of the singing voice. In most cases, it takes at least two months to adjust to the new acoustic or physical sensation created by the removal. For example, a singer with big adenoids may get lazy with raising the soft palate, because he doesn't have to lift it very high to close off the nasal pharynx. After the removal of such large obstructions, such a singer would have to retrain to use more effort to close it off. Removing the uvula (**uvulectomy**), part of the tongue (partial glossectomy), or any portion of the soft palate to correct sleep apnea or snoring is very much a last resort for singers. Surgeries that try to correct snoring are frequently unsuccessful and will definitely alter the sound of the voice due to significant alterations of the resonating cavity. Only when the singer's health is severely compromised, by insufficient oxygenation or cancerous lesions, for example, are these aggressive solutions discussed. Otherwise, other options should be discussed first, such as weight loss if being overweight is a contributing factor, for instance. As always, when you are considering treatment for your health issues, consult a medical expert. Be sure to stress that you rely heavily on your voice for your livelihood, and weigh all the options for yourself.

12.2 POSTOPERATION CONCERNS

Voice rest

Voice rest and voice conservation allow the vocal mechanism to heal after surgery. Opinions regarding appropriate amounts of voice rest vary. There is no standard voice rest treatment, and sufficient length of time differs between surgeon, condition, and patient. Laryngologists generally recommend that singers who have had vocal fold lesions removed stay completely quiet for three to no longer than fourteen days. Five days is usually a sufficient healing time for the epithelium (**re-epithelialization**) and is not so long that you'll substantially weaken the vocal muscles. It is crucial to avoid all throat clearing, coughing, and vomiting during voice rest. If you are finding it difficult to control these behaviors, contact your otolaryngologist immediately for help before more vocal damage is done.

After the period of voice rest, the singer should exercise voice conservation to avoid furthering complications with muscular atrophy. Voice conservation involves a gradual increase in voice use over the ensuing weeks. The patient should be coached before surgery on how to conserve the voice effectively so that when this period begins, talking and volume are appropriately limited and hard glottal onsets and throat clears are avoided.

The voice tends to sound better immediately following a phonosurgery, and you may be tempted to use the voice more than you should. You may also be very tempted to hear your voice because you probably have not sung much since the pathology occurred that led to the surgery in the first place. Remember, though, that your folds are still healing and are vulnerable and susceptible to injury for the first two months following surgery. The recovery from surgery is just as important as the procedure in ensuring the desired outcome. The recovery needs to be monitored very closely and under the supervision of an experienced speech-language pathologist. This involves frequent visits and imaging of the vocal folds during the first six weeks following surgery. Light scales can usually be started around four weeks after surgery. Singing is permitted once vibration returns to the vocal folds as determined by a video laryngeal stroboscopy (VLS) of the vocal folds. In most cases, singing can begin six to eight weeks after surgery, but performing is not recommended until three months after surgery, assuming appropriate rates of healing.

Note: A study has shown that a period of complete silence following vocal fold surgery doesn't hasten recovery and seven to ten days of voice conservation proves as effective as absolute voice rest. However, subjects were not singers and what is optimal to regain vocal range was not considered.

James A. Koufman and P. David Blalock. "Is Voice Rest Never Indicated?" *Journal of Voice* 3, no. 1 (1989): 87–91.

Note: A wise surgeon will take a picture of his patient's newly repaired folds immediately following the surgery. The picture is proof of their improved state and can be used later to reveal whether the patient has complied with voice rest recommendations. If the patient has not complied, follow-up pictures will likely show further damage.

Trauma-induced laryngeal web

If both vocal folds have been operated on near the anterior commissure, there is a risk of the two sides healing together and forming a laryngeal web. (See 10.13 Laryngeal Web.) The endotracheal tube often irritates vocal fold tissues as it passes through them during intubation and can also irritate as it rests in the interarytenoid space during surgery. Occasionally during long surgeries, the tube can rub the vocal folds raw or make them ulcerated. During the healing process after surgery, the sides may heal together, resulting in a web that narrows the airway and diminishes vocal quality.

Because the endotracheal tube lies in the airway, intubation irritation can occur in the trachea as well and result in a tracheal web. A web in the trachea can narrow the windpipe enough to limit airflow to the vocal folds, weakening the strength of the voice. (See Intubation in 12.1 Aspects of the Surgical Process That Concern Singers.)

Speedy recovery

Although aging and postoperative complications are out of your control, you can help healing by optimizing that which is in your control—adequate nutrition, hydration, exercise (circulation), and rest (endocrine function)—several weeks before surgery. This will prepare and equip your body to readily heal itself. (See Voice Rest in 12.2 Postoperation Concerns.)

12.3 COMMON PROBLEMS WHERE SURGERY COULD AFFECT THE VOCAL MECHANISM

Tonsillitis

When removing tonsils (tonsillectomy), care must be taken to preserve the anterior and posterior tonsillar pillars, as well as underlying musculature in the tonsillar bed. A good surgeon chooses his cuts carefully, knowing that scar tissue will form wherever he operates. The soft palate needs to be able to rise to close off the velopharyngeal port, which is the entrance into the nasopharynx. A scar in the soft palate may stiffen and tether the tissue enough that too much air escapes into the nose during phonation, causing hypernasality.

Many times an electrocautery tool called a Bovie (a.k.a. "hotstick") is used to remove tonsils. The Bovie looks like a pen with a long cord attached to a machine of controls. The Bovie functions by burning its way through tissue with electric pulses controlled at variable frequencies; the faster the electric pulse is, the deeper and more knife-like the "cutting" power. The heat of the Bovie seals off (cauterizes) blood vessels as it burns. However, two other techniques are preferred over the Bovie when removing singers' tonsils. One technique is to use the clean precise cuts of a knife and scissors followed with stitches to stop the bleeding. This method uses no heat and causes less scarring than electrocauterization. The other preferred method uses radiofrequency to dissect the tonsils. Radiofrequency uses much less heat than the Bovie and therefore does less thermal damage to the tissues surrounding what it "cuts" so there's less scarring.

Ovarian surgery

Operations on the ovaries change endocrine production and can lead to hormonal imbalance. Side effects include a decrease in range, hoarseness, masculinization of the female voice, and other alterations in vocal color. These changes can be decreased by the use of hormone replacement therapy. Beware of pituitary brain surgery, which can also change the hormonal balance in the body and cause these side effects.

Cesarean section and hysterectomy

All laparotomies (large abdominal wall incisions) affect respiratory musculature and take six to twelve weeks to heal. (See Respiratory Alteration in 12.1 Aspects of the Surgical Process That Concern Singers.) Six weeks following abdominal surgery, ten- to fifteen-minute periods of monitored daily vocalizing should commence. Gradually increase frequency and intensity. Presurgery levels of singing will not be reached until abdominal muscles have completely healed. Reconditioning may take up to two years postoperation.

Wisdom teeth removal

Voice use will be very difficult for several weeks after having wisdom teeth removed due to oral swelling and painful jaw movement. These effects are temporary and should resolve with healing. However, your orthodontist must take care during any orthodontic procedure to not hyperextend your jaw. The jaw can dislocate and develop a temporomandibular joint disorder disruptive to singing. (See **temporomandibular joint disorder** in 15.3 Vocabulary.)

Sleep apnea

Sleep apnea is a very common problem that can cause uvula and soft palate hypertrophy and lead to more serious long-term medical issues such as heart disease, high blood pressure, reflux, and breathing difficulties. There is no way to surgically correct sleep apnea in a singer without affecting the voice. **Uvulopalatopharyngoplasty** or "**UP3**" includes the removal of the uvula (**uvulectomy**) and portions of the soft palate, as well as possibly stiffening the soft palate with inserts to prevent snoring. Other corrective measures include removing the tonsils, portions of the nasal structures, or tongue (partial glossectomy). The radical alteration to the articulators and resonating cavities would be devastating to the singing voice and has only a 50% success rate for correcting the apnea. A much safer and more successful treatment is available using a device known as a continuous positive airway pressure (CPAP) mask. The air pressure prevents the collapse of tissues that cause the apnea. This device uses a facial mask, nasal mask, or nasal inserts to deliver the positive pressure. This method is virtually 100% successful in reversing sleep apnea.

Vocal fold medial edge lesions

Unless cancer or an unresolvable pathology deems otherwise, singers are rarely candidates for microlaryngeal surgery, simply because any surgery performed on the folds disrupts the cover to some degree. A lesion occurring anywhere along the vocal folds' medial edge is most problematic, because the edges must be smooth and unscarred to vibrate periodically and produce a pure tone.

Medial edge surface lesions (e.g., nodules) respond well to expert therapy, and surgery is a risky last resort. Removal methods involve stripping a portion of the folds or grabbing the lesion with 30-degree upward biting cupped forceps ("up cups") or straight biting forceps and tearing it away from the rest of the fold. (See 12.5 Common Instruments and Materials Used in Microlaryngeal Surgery.) Both methods leave the medial edge irreparably scarred to the point of possible dysphonia and even aphonia. If the medial edge lesion is superficial (e.g., a polyp) or subepithelial (e.g., a cyst) and does not respond to therapy, a special surgical technique can be employed to ensure preservation of the medial vibrating edge. This technique involves cutting lateral to the folds' medial edge and working under the cover layer. When the surgery is complete, the cover flap is relaid and the precious vibrating edges are left undisturbed. Even when the medial edge is successfully preserved, however, the healing that takes place beneath the surface will still diminish vocal function to some degree.

12.4 MICROLARYNGEAL SURGERY

Microlaryngeal surgery is a relatively noninvasive method of operating (because you are not cut open) on the larynx in which the surgeon operates with specially designed instruments that he feeds into your mouth and down your pharynx via a metal scope (operating laryngoscope) while peering through a microscopic lens that magnifies the larynx. Accessing the larynx in this way is helpful in obtaining a biopsy from the larynx to rule out cancer. When the goal is to improve voice quality, whether it is removing a lesion on the vocal fold or injecting a substance to bulk the vocal fold, microlaryngeal surgery is referred to as phonosurgery and is *the* surgery of choice.

12.5 COMMON INSTRUMENTS AND MATERIALS USED IN
MICROLARYNGEAL SURGERY

The mouthguard, also known as the mouthpiece, is like that of a football player and protects the teeth from the metal laryngoscope. (See Figure 12.5a.) The mouthguard is used to minimize the risk of chipping the teeth during the surgery. Singers would be wise to have a mouthguard custom made for them by their dentist—just to keep on hand. Even buying a drug store mouthguard that can be warmed and molded to the mouth will fit better than the one-size-fits-all mouthguard used in the operating room. The type of metal scope used for operating will vary between patients. Experienced laryngeal surgeons have between five and ten scopes to choose from when performing vocal fold surgery. The scopes vary in name, length, width, and shape. When determining which scope will offer the best visibility, the surgeon will consider whether he will be operating on the posterior or anterior end of the vocal fold and take into account the shape of the patient's throat. (Generally a smaller and shorter scope is used for females.) If undergoing surgery, be sure your laryngologist has at least four scope options. Occasionally several scopes may be used on the same patient to accomplish the surgery. The scope is passed into the mouth, over the tongue, and down the neck, stopping just before the false folds.

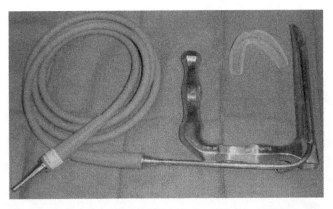

Figure 12.5a The Mouthguard, Operating Laryngoscope, and Light Source

Unlike nasendoscopes and oral endoscopes used in the clinic for exams, the operating scopes don't magnify. They are merely hollow pipes with openings along the sides for a light tube, camera, and suction to pass through. The surgeon peers through the scope with a high-powered microscope used to magnify and improve the visualization of the vocal folds while operating. The light source (blue cord) inserts into the scope and filters a bright light through its tube. Bright halogen lighting is required to perform the surgery. This magnification and bright lighting allow him to clearly see where to make incisions and help him to isolate the cover of the vocal fold so he can avoid damaging it. Pressure from the operating laryngoscope resting on the tongue during surgery can cause a temporary distortion of, or temporary loss of, taste sensation. This generally resolves within two to three weeks.

The laryngoscope is held in position by a suspension device so that the physician has both hands free to operate. The suspension supports and steadies the scope by anchoring it to the instrument table over the patient.

Long-handled instruments with tiny operative tips are fed into the operating laryngoscope to perform fine detail work in the larynx. Scissor-like handles are used to control the mechanics of the small tool at the tip. (See Figures 12.5b and 12.5c.) With the help

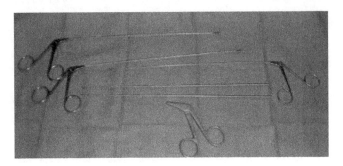

Figure 12.5b Microinstruments
Microinstruments are operated with scissor-like handles.

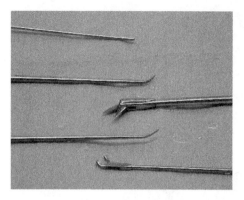

FIGURE 12.5c Microinstrument Tips
The microinstruments do fine detail work. From top to bottom:
The laryngeal probe has a blunt tip, used to move tissue out of the way for examination.
The elevator flap is used to lift tissue.
The up-scissors or 45-degree angle scissors are used to separate tissue and dissect.
The sickle knife makes straight, clean incisions, otherwise known as microflaps.
The 30-degree upward biting cupped forceps may be used to grab and pull tissue out of the way. This action is known as retraction. Straight biting cupped forceps may be used in their place, depending on the surgeon's preference.

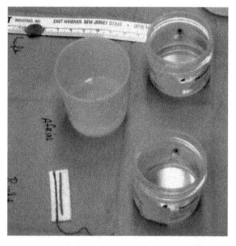

FIGURE 12.5d Cottonoid, Afrin®, Formalin, and Specimen
Cottonoids (7 o'clock) are manufactured on a string that is oft en colored for easy landmarking and accessibility during use. Afrin, a form of adrenaline (center). Formalin (2 and 4 o'clock) is a toxic preservative and is used to store the specimens that will be taken to the lab for testing following the surgery. A large specimen of polypoid tissue (on ruler) has been removed in one neat, self-contained piece.

of magnifying lenses, the physician is able to use a variety of tips to accomplish minute retractions, incisions, and biopsies.

A cottonoid may be fed with forceps into the laryngoscope to swab blood around the area of operation. Often the cottonoid is first soaked in an **adrenaline** solution to help contract and shrink blood vessels. The adrenaline solution makes for a less messy surgery and offers more visibility for deciphering anatomy and cutting. Cups of a formaldehyde solution are used for any tissue that is removed and needs to be preserved for further examination in the hospital lab.

13

A Hypothetical Microlaryngeal Phonosurgery

WHILE SOME OF the details regarding scheduling and clinic protocols may vary slightly from center to center, this chapter explains what to expect during a voice surgery. This step-by-step account of an actual vocal fold polyp surgery takes you from check-in, onto the gurney and into the operating room, continuing through what's happening while you're asleep until you wake up postoperation and begin your recovery at home.

13.1 SCHEDULING

After determining that your pathology is not going to resolve with therapy, surgical intervention may be necessary. Because the recovery period is just as important as the operation for regaining optimal voice, the timing of your surgery is important. The physician discusses the procedure with you as well as his postoperative expectations, such as length of rest and when to return to work and resume normal activities. You express all your concerns and fears and choose a date that allows you to comply with postoperative demands. A follow-up is scheduled as well for one week following the surgery.

> Note: Remember to choose a surgery time when your selected anesthesiologist is available as well.

13.2 CHECK-IN

You check in one to two hours prior to your operation and meet with a secretary to fill out paperwork. You assure the secretary that you've prepared your gastrointestinal tract for general anesthesia by refraining from food and liquids, other than water, for the last eight hours.

13.3 PREOPERATIVE CARE

You are assigned and led to a room where you remove all jewelry, make-up, and clothing and don an ID bracelet, hospital gown, and robe. Personal items are bagged, labeled, and stored in a postoperative area locker. You lie covered up on a bed in a preoperative waiting area. You're asked to state any product and medication allergies or sensitivities. A registered nurse inserts an intravenous (IV) line into the back of your hand and fluids are delivered into your bloodstream to keep the vein open and replace any fluid that is missing in your body.

> Note: The hand tends to be the easiest area on the body to see veins and is more comfortable than the inner part of the arm opposite the elbow where blood samples are commonly drawn. The inner wrist is very uncomfortable and used as a last resort. The jugular vein in the neck is used for big operations like heart or lung surgeries.

You are then wheeled to the operating room where your bed is parked with the head of the bed toward the anesthesiologist. As a precaution, teeth are checked and imperfections noted so the hospital has a record in the unlikely case that further damage is done. The anesthesiologist puts an oxygen mask over your mouth and asks you to breathe deeply to ensure that your oxygen levels are high before administering medication. He monitors your vital signs and warns you that you might feel a burning sensation in your hand as he drips a hypnotic sedative into your IV line (e.g., Versed', a short-acting Valium'-like drug). He asks that you keep breathing. This premedication calms you and creates an amnesia-like effect so that you remember little afterward. He adds a general anesthesia drug to the drip (e.g., Pentothal' or propofol).[1] The drug takes immediate effect. Your face muscles twitch involuntarily and then fall slack. Now that you're asleep, the anesthesiologist drips a muscle relaxant medication into the IV to release your jaw for the endotracheal tube insertion. He fits a mouthguard over your teeth and then looks with a lighted intubating laryngoscope into your mouth to spray your folds with lidocaine. Finally, sure that the muscle relaxation has taken full effect, he inserts the endotracheal tube through your mouth and into your pharynx to rest between the folds.

Gauging its depth by the centimeter markings on the tube in reference to your teeth, he stops once it's a few centimeters beyond your vocal folds and in the upper third of your trachea. The tube is then taped to the left side of your mouth so that the laryngoscope can be fitted **centrally**. Attached to a machine-run pump, the tube feeds air and anesthesia gas in and out of your lungs, maintaining your normal breathing while keeping you asleep. The bed is turned so that your head is now toward the physician.

---

[1] Anesthesiologist, Dr. Kenneth P. Gross, e-mail message to author, January 7, 2011.

13.4 THE OPERATION

Scrubbed to the elbows, and masked and dressed by a scrub tech, the laryngolo-gist enters the operating room. He asks that a pillow be placed under your neck to allow your head to drop back. He moves your tongue to one side and slides the rigid laryngoscope straight into your mouth, through the oropharynx and stopping just short of the laryngopharynx at the epiglottis or **vallecula** for a direct view of the glottis. The scope is anchored to the instrument table by a suspension. The physi-cian runs the light cord down the outside right of the scope until the vocal folds are illuminated. The light actually causes the outside of your neck to glow red. The bed is lowered and the physician sits in a chair just behind and level with your head. (See Figures 13.4a and 13.4b.) He peers down the scope's tunnel through magnifying lenses and takes preoperative pictures. These pictures are printed and inserted into your chart by a technician.

The physician then inserts a skinny, long-handled pair of straight biting forceps down the scope and gently grasps the polyp to expose and stabilize the area to be cut. (See Figure 13.4c.) Your folds twitch against the forceps, and he orders the anesthesi-ologist to increase the muscle relaxant, which has a paralysis-like effect on the folds.

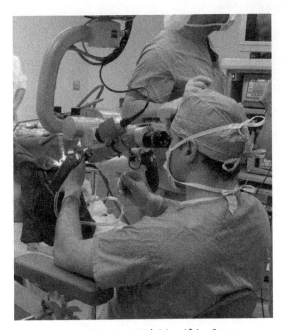

FIGURE 13.4a Operating With Magnifying Lenses
The laryngologist is seated at the patient's head (covered for picture to protect identity). He is peering into the operat-ing laryngoscope using magnifying lenses and inserting a microinstrument into the operating laryngoscope to perform phonosurgery.

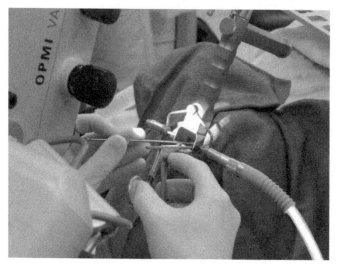

FIGURE 13.4b Operating via Laryngoscope With Microinstruments
Notice glowing light cord inserted along right side of operating laryngoscope to illuminate larynx. This laryngoscope, light source tube, and microinstrument are similar but different models than those pictured in Figure 12.5a.

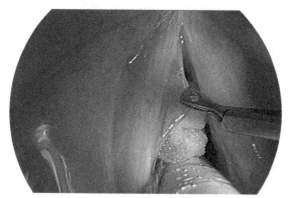

FIGURE 13.4c Magnified Lesion and Intubation Tube
Straight biting forceps are used to grasp the polyp and expose the area alongside it for a precise lateral cut. An Afrin -soaked cottonoid (see blue string and cottonoid also pictured in Figure 12.5d) helps to shrink blood vessels and make for a less gory process.

He uses tiny scissors to cut into the epithelium immediately alongside the medial edge and moves carefully under the epithelium, gently exposing the polypoid lesion. He checks his scissors' location under the loosened tissue, making sure as he cuts that the vocal ligament is behind the scissors. (See Figure 13.4d.) Left vocal fold lesions are easier for right-handed people to operate on, and the physician permits his observing resident to remove the polyp.

The resident carefully moves the scissor blade under the thin layer of epithelium, being cautious to cut, not tear it. Some of the epithelium is extremely thin from being stretched around a lesion. Stretched-out, floppy tissue isn't good anymore and any part of it that doesn't run along the medial edge of the fold is removed for neat healing.

Because the tissue is redundant and damaged, removing it will not leave a gap when the epithelium heals but will help maintain a smooth vibrating edge. The excised tissue is handed to the scrub technician, who promptly seals the specimen in a cup of **formalin** to be taken to the lab for testing. The physician soaks a cottonoid in Afrin´ and feeds it down the scope to swab blood from your folds and constrict the blood vessels. Pictures are taken of your folds. (See Figure 13.4e.)

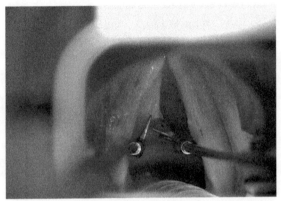

FIGURE 13.4d Magnified Cutting of Lesion
Using scissors to cut lateral to the vibrating edge allows precise cutting into the lesion and removal of damaged tissue with little alteration to the medial edge.

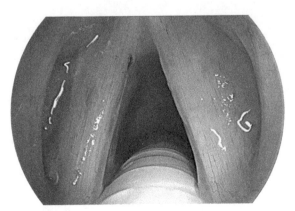

Figure 13.4e Magnified Folds Postexcision
Only the damaged tissue has been removed from the right vocal fold and the mucosal layer is re-laid. Note the near-normal appearance of the vocal fold edge. The vibrating edge has been preserved as much as possible.

The "before and after shots" are filed in your chart for future reference. Doubles are made for your personal use and are given to the nurse so that he may give them to you after you wake up. The surgeon tells the anesthesiologist that the operation will be done soon and preparations are made to help you wake up.

13.5 POSTOPERATIVE CARE

As the anesthesia gas starts to wear off, you begin to breathe on your own and wake up, gagging a lot as you come down from the drugs. The anesthesiologist used a lot of muscle relaxant and had to compensate with another medication to reverse its effects and get your muscles to respond faster. (This routine is not uncommon.) Your stomach and abdominal muscles ache and your neck is sore from surgical intubation, extubation, and the operating laryngoscope positioning. A couple of scrub technicians move you onto a new clean bed and wheel you to a room of monitored recovering patients. Here, you fully wake up as the nurse drapes a prewarmed flannel blanket over you and aims heat lamps at your body.[2] The anesthesia caused your body's temperature to drop and your body shivers, trying to regulate itself. Your shivering doesn't even compare to the patient across from you who had open-heart surgery and shivers from a much more significant loss of body heat. (Phonosurgery is comparatively noninvasive and rarely causes a body's temperature to drop in and of itself.) You gesture to the nurse for something to write with, because you must begin your five-day voice rest observance. You want to clear your throat, but you realize that voice rest means no clearing, coughing, sneezing, and whispering. Instead, you gesture for some ice chips. You sleep. The nurse determines that your vital signs have normalized and you are wheeled to a postoperative room where you rest and wait for your ride home.

Note: Occasionally, stomach and abdominal muscles ache after general anesthesia. The reason for the ache, called postoperative myalgia, is not clear, but it is generally attributed to the uncoordinated tensing of muscles that occurs with the administering of some muscle relaxants just before relaxation takes effect. The ache seems to occur more frequently in women, particularly those who receive a muscle relaxant called succinylcholine. The ache usually resolves after two to three days.

---

[2] Many operating facilities use a forced warm air gown before, during, and after surgery to help keep the body's temperature normal.

13.6 AT HOME

You don't use your voice at all for three whole days. On the fourth day, you speak softly for about five minutes every hour but are careful to resist the urge to cough or clear your throat. Every other day you increase the time you talk by about five minutes. Your voice is unpredictable and pitch is very difficult to control, making you sound like a pubescent boy. These pitch breaks will last about three to four weeks. After the fourth week you may be allowed to resume singing a little. The best healing you can hope for as a singer is about 95% of your normal voice. You still can't taste the food you eat and won't be able to until the four weeks are up due to the pressure the metal scope put on your tongue. Your jaw, throat, and tongue feel bruised but are no longer in pain. The bruised feeling will go away in just a couple weeks.

14

Common Questions Answered

THE FIFTEEN QUESTIONS answered in this chapter are frequently asked and were collected from college-aged singers and actors.

14.1 WHAT GIVES US EACH OUR OWN UNIQUE SOUND?

It's important to realize that if you took the larynx out of your body and were able to get the vocal folds to vibrate, the sound would be a pretty generic buzz. The pitch of the buzz would vary, depending on slight differences in the length and thickness of the vocal folds, but the fundamental size and shape of your resonating cavities are what really distinguish your voice. The buzzing sound at the vocal fold level resonates in the spaces above that make up the vocal tract. Your laryngeal vestibule, pharynx, and oral cavity are the resonators that influence your voice quality the most, but your nose and sinus cavities contribute to your sound as well.

Except pitch and loudness, voice quality refers to all the characteristics of your sound such as resonance (e.g., nasal, oral, forward ping), timbre (warm), and color (e.g., bright, dark, brassy). Within your physical limitations, you have an amazing ability to manipulate your voice's natural quality by changing the shape of your resonators (nasal cavities, oral cavity, and pharynx). For instance, you can sound more nasal by relaxing your soft palate, thus allowing some of your buzzing sound to resonate in the nasal cavity. Contracting your aryepiglottic sphincter in your laryngopharynx while lowering your soft palate in your oral cavity will give you a bright witch's cackle. Or you can sound more operatic by raising the soft palate (as in the beginning of a yawn) so that it closes off the nasopharynx and redirects your buzzing sound out the oral cavity only. Protruding your lips elongates the oral cavity and can darken your sound.

14.2 WHY DOES MY RECORDED VOICE SOUND DIFFERENT?

When we listen to ourselves, our ears are not only picking up the sound that leaves our mouth but also picking up the sound through our interior physiology (bone conduction). If we plug our ears, we can still hear our voice, but the sound is dampened from the bone, liquid, and tissue of our skulls. This dampening lessens the accuracy with which we perceive our own voices. The voice on tape does not match what those around you are accustomed to hearing either! Healthy ears hear a very broad sound spectrum, whereas electronic recording devices encompass a limited gamut of the sound spectrum, usually clipping upper-frequency peaks, and thus deadening the overall brilliance of tone. The broader the frequency range is in a recorder, microphone, and so forth, the closer you'll come to hearing yourself accurately. Many digital recording devices today simulate a near-perfect likeness.

14.3 HOW ARE OPERA SINGERS HEARD OVER AN ORCHESTRA WITHOUT AMPLIFICATION?

It's not just opera singers! While opera singers are specifically trained so that their voices can be heard over an orchestra without any use of amplification, this acoustic advantage is available to singers of other genres of music and even speakers. Acoustics computer programs are available that provide visual feedback as you sing or speak in order to help you develop this "ringy" sound.

You can think of the vocal tract as a 16.3-cm-long (6.4-inch-long) tube, closed at the vocal fold end and open at the mouth (and nose) end.[1] This tube has harmonic peaks around 500, 1,500, 2,500, and 3,500 Hz, meaning that when the vocal folds vibrate 500 cycles in a second (cps), the frequency complements the space and resonates louder. No other instrument can produce harmonic peaks at 2,500 Hz or higher. An orchestra's frequency peaks at about 450 Hz. Because our ears reach peak resonance at about 3,000 Hz, singers and speakers who

---

Note: The boost or peak in the energy of the voice varies somewhat depending on whether you're speaking or singing and what voice type you are. A bass will have a lower frequency peak than a soprano, for example. The estimated range of **hertz** in voice science literature varies somewhat. The studies don't always specify voice types, and some only test actors while others only analyze belters or classical singers. Everyone's peak falls somewhere between 2,000 Hz and 4,000 Hz, regardless of voice type, speaking, or singing.

---

[1] Steve An Xue and Jianping G. Hao, "Normative Standards for Vocal Tract Dimensions by Race as Measured by Acoustic Pharyngometry," *Journal of Voice* 20, no. 3 (September 2006): 391–400. (Measured from glottis to lip)

are able to consistently produce a harmonic peak or a "ring" at around 2,500 to 3,500 Hz while they phonate have an acoustical advantage and do not need electrical amplification.

Singers who study Western classical singing technique focus on mastering this ringing voice quality some have referred to as "mask resonance" (because it produces vibrations felt in the face bones), "*squillo*," or the **Singer's Formant**. (See Sympathetic "Resonance" in 9.5 Misnomers.)

There is some controversy about what is physically happening to produce this boost in spectral energy. Many theories have been proposed, and it may be that we discover there is more than one way to achieve it. Many believe that it is the narrowing or contraction of the aryepiglottic sphincter. This narrowed effect essentially creates a resonator within a resonator and may result in this dramatically brighter sound. (See **laryngeal tube** and **aryepiglottic sphincter** in 15.3 Vocabulary.) Many consider the Singer's Formant to be specific to classical singers and have come to equate it with the operatic sound. In actuality, the same formant can be heard in some country singers and is referred to as twang. It's also produced by a lot of healthy belters who call it brass. The Singer's Formant in operatic singing may not seem as *perceptually* bright as belting or twang, because opera singers balance or warm the potentially "brassy" brightness by singing with the larynx in a slightly lower position. Opera singers' combination breathing involves relaxing the abdominal muscles, which actually helps to draw the larynx into this lower position. Belting, which tends to involve more chest-dominant breath, couples a slightly higher larynx with more thyroarytenoid muscle contraction, which makes for a very bright and heavy quality. Country singing tends to involve a higher laryngeal position and more fold mass as well. Squillo, twang, brass—all have carrying power over an orchestra. Because articles are being written on the "*Speaker's Formant*" that refer to the same spectral boost in energy, we feel that a more inclusive term than "Singer's Formant" is needed, one that is free of aesthetic connotations. "Twang" tends to be associated with a southern dialect or bluegrass music. "Brassy" carries a negative connotation among classical singers. We'd like to propose that "Rocket Formant" might be a good replacement because of the powerful boost this resonance adds to the voice.[2]

14.4 HOW DO I AVOID GETTING NODULES?

Hydrate; don't talk too loudly, too much, or too low; warm up the voice in the morning before beginning to speak; speak on the breath, inflecting and maintaining tone to the ends of sentences; warm up properly before singing; avoid pressing or straining to speak or sing; control reflux if you have it. Any sensation felt in the neck while singing or talking suggests constriction and is a good sign that you're doing something inefficiently. Prenodular conditions can resolve with one or two days of voice rest or conservation and good hydration. (See 10.5 Vocal Fold Nodules.)

---

[2] Kerrie Obert, CCC-SLP, coined this term.

You don't have a separate speaking voice and a separate singing voice. You have one voice. Even if you're not a singer but have difficulty with the way you speak, consider taking singing lessons and applying what you learn to optimize the efficiency of your speaking.

Here is a quick "Masterclass for the Speaking Voice":

Stand like you do to sing: bend side to side, lifting out of your hips; elongate upward through the back of the neck; anchor yourself on the floor so it would be hard for someone to push you over. Feel very east–west through the chest and shoulder blades.

Begin humming with just the inner portion of your lips touching—do this until your lips really tickle and you feel mask vibrations.

Find your optimal speaking tessitura by humming with your ears plugged. (See note on optimal speaking tessitura in 3.9 Vocal Hazards.)

Take a breath without feeling like you are holding tension anywhere. Be conscious of not holding your breath before you begin to speak, but use inhalation like the wind-up before throwing a ball and speak right away.

Speak on a sufficient amount of breath in order to keep tone in every word—right to the end of your sentences.

Vary the inflection in your speech

Maintain the same mask vibrations (a.k.a. forward focus) that you use for singing.

14.5 WHAT ARE THE BEST/WORST TYPES OF BEVERAGES FOR MY VOICE AROUND PERFORMANCES?

Water is the beverage of choice. Beware of alcohol, caffeine, and carbonated beverages. (See 3.4 Foods to Avoid and Why.)

14.6 SHOULD I REALLY AVOID DAIRY PRODUCTS WHILE IN PRODUCTION?

To digest fatty dairy products, the body must produce viscous mucus that helps break it down for digestion. To avoid singing with thick mucus, allow yourself an hour and a half to digest after consuming dairy before singing. (See 3.4 Foods to Avoid and Why.)

14.7 HOW MUCH TIME SHOULD I SPEND WARMING UP BEFORE A LESSON?

You know your voice better than anyone else. The time it takes to achieve that warmed-up feeling varies with each individual. During the run of a show, singers may stay warmed up and need only ten minutes, when normally they might need half an hour to feel ready vocally. The amount of time needed to warm up may depend on the time of the day, the time of the month for some women, when and what you last ate, and the level of difficulty in what you're about to sing. Learn to recognize when you feel warmed up and what it took you to get there. Remember, it's called "warming up," not "beautiful singing," so don't beat yourself up or force the voice if the first few sounds you make are substandard. Be very careful not to oversing or rush into your extreme top and bottom ranges. Begin by "warming" your easiest sounds in your most comfortable range. Keep in mind that the reason you warm up the voice is to be able to sing your loudest, softest, highest, and lowest without strain.

14.8   WHAT EXACTLY HAPPENS WHEN MY VOICE GETS HOARSE?

Hoarseness is a combination of excessive air leaking through the vocal folds as they phonate (because the folds are not entirely closed), vocal fold stiffness (due to a lesion or vocal fold swelling), and pressed or constricted laryngeal muscles. The result is often a tight, raspy sound. The folds must be hydrated, have smooth edges (i.e., no lesions), and be uniform in weight (i.e., no hemorrhaged blood vessels) in order to have the periodic cover wave that produces what we recognize as a clean sound.

14.9   WHAT HAPPENS WHEN I LOSE MY VOICE?

Also known as aphonia, having no voice usually implies acute inflammation. (See 10.2 Laryngitis.) The folds become so swollen that they are weighed down and stiff. Vibration is absent or severely decreased, irregular, and slow. More phonatory pressure and increased breath flow is needed to initiate a tone. If you have to push to get a tone started, something is wrong. In such cases, voice rest is better than phonation.

14.10   WHAT CAUSES VIBRATO?

Is vibrato taught, imitated, or inherent? Is it voluntary or involuntary? Is it a natural or contrived vocal characteristic? The finest vocal pedagogues, pathologists, and performers debate these questions, but the issue remains unresolved. Three main theories exist:

   Vibrato is muscularly produced and manipulatively controlled.
   Vibrato is learned and/or imitated.
   Vibrato is an organic, natural phenomenon.

We believe vibrato may be explained by all three theories. In different classically trained singers' video laryngeal stroboscopy (VLS) exams, we've observed how visually varied vibrato appears. Any number of laryngeal structures may shake: sometimes the soft palate, the back of the tongue, the pharyngeal walls, or the larynx itself, and other times two or three of these combined.

Vibrato may occur from a slight letting go or lowering of muscular effort, with overly relaxed laryngeal musculature producing an out-of-control vibrato and held laryngeal muscular effort straightening the tone.[3] The mystery remains, however, as to what exactly is being relaxed and what exactly is being contracted.

14.11 TO WHAT EXTENT IS A GREAT VOICE DETERMINED BY VOCAL PHYSIOLOGY?

A great voice is a combination of natural-born physiology, training, and musical instinct. Aside from the slight length and width variant that generally distinguish a male's vocal folds from a female's, all vocal folds are essentially alike. It's a person's ability to coordinate his or her breath and vocal folds and that person's resonator shapes and sizes, as well as his or her ability to be musical, that factor into a beautiful voice. In other words, if you could somehow exchange your own larynx with Renee Fleming's, your voice may sound slightly different, but still not like hers due to your unique oral, nasal, laryngeal, and pharyngeal cavities. Even if you were to have Renee Fleming's exact anatomical structure but still have your brain controlling the muscular motion, you would not be able to sing like her. Our voices, like every other part of us, are wired up to our brain. Two people singing along with the radio may produce very different perceptions depending on what their brains do with the information they're receiving. One person may consistently sing a whole tone lower than the song they're hearing, while another may occasionally go slightly sharp or flat but maintain relative accuracy. It's safe to say that every healthy person is able to improve his or her voice and learn to sing.

14.12 WHAT CAUSES A TICKLE?

Usually a tickle occurs with infection (e.g., the common cold), irritation (e.g., dust, laryngopharyngeal reflux [LPR]), or dehydration of the larynx. We've even noticed that the superficial dryness triggered by a nervous adrenaline rush seems to cause a tickle. Tensing and constricting laryngeal muscles during phonation can also create an itchy or tickly sensation as the vocal folds are slammed together and their freedom to vibrate is limited.

---

[3] The author assumes vibrato to be what generally pleases the Western ear, five to seven pulsations per second.

14.13 MY VOICE GETS SO TIRED WHEN I'M TRYING
TO MEMORIZE MUSIC. WHAT SHOULD I DO?

Singing a song over and over is not the most efficient or effective way to memorize a piece of music. You want to sing songs when your voice is fresh and strong. Singing a song over and over may help stick it in your muscle memory, but if the voice is tired, your muscle memory could be memorizing bad habits that often accompany tired vocal production as well. It's much more efficient to learn your music through means other than your voice. Memorizing can be very quick and more effective when varied approaches are applied to learning a given piece. I—the primary author of this book—have found that the songs I memorized through repetitive singing only are the ones that have escaped me in performance. There is nothing worse than being on stage and having no idea what word is sung next and no logical way of getting it to come to you, other than singing a phrase over or moving on to a later section. The following approaches allow me to memorize efficiently and thoroughly while saving my voice. The best part of this process is how expressive and alive I'm free to be when I finally perform a piece learned in this way:

If a recording is available, listen to it once to grasp the general style and tradition of the piece. Don't learn a piece by listening to a recording, or your personal artistic creativity will suffer.

If the text is in another language, translate it literally word for word.

Decipher the poetic sense of the text and write out every sentence in your own words. Do this even if you already have a poetic translation available. (You can use www.babelfish.com/ if you get stumped.)

Write the text (in the sung language) on a piece of paper. Look for patterns, such as repetitive lines, and break it up into sections.

Choosing a section of the text, stick the paper in your pocket and take a walk, going over that section and referring to the paper as needed. Speak it, sing it under your breath, or just lip sync it. Do this during mundane tasks such as showering, washing dishes, and riding in the car. Avoid constantly building off the beginning so that the beginning is overlearned and the end is never as polished.

Write the text out again and again from memory, referring to the paper in your pocket as needed.

Give the paper to someone else and have him or her test your memorization.

Learn the music of the song and put it with the text. Study the composer's choices for the musical expression of the text. Pay attention to what the dynamics, melody, harmonies, and accompaniment are doing when you sing the text. Is it mirroring the feelings expressed?

Speak the text as though it's a story or monologue. Decide to whom you're talking and experiment to discover new ways of expressing the text. Continue this process as you go on to the next approach.

Now sing it with good technique and all the nuances, emotions, and colors you found throughout the memorization process. Your performance is likely to be more unique and expressive. And if you forget a word, though it will be less likely, your brain will have many ways of recalling it.

14.14 WHAT DO MY VOCAL FOLDS LOOK LIKE WHEN I SING A WHISTLE TONE?

Also known as the female falsetto or flute register, whistle tone occurs when the folds are elongated to their longest and thinnest. The folds approximate as though to phonate, but never quite make contact. Because the folds do not touch, they never go through a closed phase when vibrating, and actual phonation doesn't occur. As the air passes between them, they produce a tiny cover wave as they flutter and essentially whistle. (Think of a reed instrument.) The folds appear slightly bowed when producing a whistle tone due to the absence of thyroarytenoid muscle contraction, which gives adducted vocal folds varying degrees of bulk. Mariah Carey is a pop singer who easily accesses whistle tones.

14.15 WHY DO SOME SINGERS FIND VOCAL AGILITY EASY AND OTHERS FIND IT MORE DIFFICULT?

There are singers who perform roulades, trills, fioratura, melismas, runs, and portamenti effortlessly. These singers' physiques vary from thin to large (compare classical sopranos like Lily Pons and Jessye Norman), their sound may be big or small, and their tessitura higher (pop singer Mariah Carey or Disney's original Snow White, Adriana Caselotti) or lower (classical mezzo soprano Cecilia Bartoli). Although it is healthy for all singers to work on their agility regularly to develop and maintain flexibility, some will reap more impressive results than others. Although very little research has been done, we speculate that a secret ingredient to being naturally predisposed to coloratura agility lies in the ratio of slow-twitch fibers to fast-twitch fibers in the thyroarytenoid muscles. Fast-twitch fibers are the muscles closest to the medial edges of the folds that allow for high-speed contraction. The vocal folds of a coloratura may tend to have more fast-twitch muscle fibers and a sharper edge to the medial vibrating lips during phonation. A lyric's vocal folds may have fewer fast-twitch fibers and slightly rounder vibrating edges during phonation.

15

Glossary

You should request copies of your medical records to have for your own personal file. In trying to decipher some of the codes you may come across in your charts or hear during a clinic visit, you may find this list helpful.

AES:	aryepiglottic sphincter
ASL:	analysis through synthesis lab
Ba:	barium
Ben:	benign
Bid:	twice a day
Bx:	biopsy
CC:	chief complaint
CCC-SLP:	Certificate of Clinical Competence in Speech-Language Pathology
C/O:	complains of
CN X:	cranial nerve #10
CNS:	central nervous system
cps:	cycles per second
dB:	decibel
D/C:	discontinue
D.O.:	doctor of osteopathy
Dx:	diagnosis
EGG:	electroglottogram
Endo:	endoscopy

ETT:	endotracheal tube
ETOH:	alcohol
FO:	fundamental frequency
FEES°:	Fiberoptic Endoscopic Evaluation of Swallowing
FFN:	flexible fiberoptic nasendoscopy
FHx:	family history
F/U:	follow-up
GE:	gastroesophageal
GERD:	gastroesophageal reflux disease
GI:	gastrointestinal
Haz-Mat:	hazardous materials, usually referring to drugs
HEENT:	head, eyes, ears, nose, and throat
HPV:	human papilloma virus
HTN:	hypertension
Hx:	history
Hz:	hertz
IC:	inspiratory capacity
Insp:	inspiration
IV:	intravenous
JAMA:	*Journal of the American Medical Association*
Ⓛ:	left
LAT:	lateral
LEHPZ:	lower esophageal high-pressure zone
LES:	lower esophageal sphincter
LO:	lateral oblique
LPR:	laryngopharyngeal reflux
LRI:	lower respiratory infection
LTB:	laryngotracheobronchitis
Memb:	membrane
ML:	midline
MP:	menstrual period
MTD:	muscle tension dysphonia
NATS:	National Association of Teachers of Singing, Inc.
NG:	nasogastric tube
NKA:	no known allergies
NL:	normal
NP:	nasopharynx
NT:	nasotracheal
Obl:	oblique
Obst:	obstruction
Occ:	occasional
O.P.C.:	outpatient clinic
OSA(S):	obstructive sleep apnea syndrome
Palp:	palpable
PC:	after meals

PEG:	percutaneous endoscopic gastrostomy
PO:	by mouth
Postop:	postoperative
Prelim:	preliminary
Preop:	preoperative
Prep:	prepare
Prim:	primary
PMS:	premenstrual syndrome
PT:	patient
PVFM:	paradoxical vocal fold movement
®:	right
RFOE:	rigid fiberoptic oral endoscopy
RLN:	recurrent laryngeal nerve
R/t:	related to
RVT:	resonant voice therapy
Rx:	prescription
SLN:	superior laryngeal nerve
SLP:	speech-language pathologist
SMR:	submucous resection
SOB:	shortness of breath
SVS:	singing voice specialist
Symp:	symptoms
T&A:	tonsillectomy and adenoidectomy (adenotonsillectomy)
TE:	tracheoesophageal
TFL:	transnasal fiberoptic laryngoscopy
TLV:	total lung volume
TMD:	temporomandibular joint dysfunction (or disorder)
TMJ:	temporomandibular joint
TPR:	temperature, pulse, and respirations
TV:	tidal volume
Tx:	treatment
UES:	upper esophageal sphincter
UGI:	upper gastrointestinal
Unk:	unknown
UPPP/UP3:	uvulopalatopharyngoplasty
URI:	upper respiratory infection
VAS:	vascular
VC:	vital capacity
VCD:	**vocal cord dysfunction**
VF:	ventricular fibrillation
Vent:	ventricle
VLS:	video laryngeal stroboscopy
Vol:	volume
VS:	vital signs
VSD:	ventricular septal defect

WNL: within normal limits
Wt: weight
X/R: x-ray

15.2 SUFFIXES

Knowing the following common suffixes may help you decipher jargon used by clinicians and physicians in the hospital and clinic.

-caine: a suffix classifying a group of **local anesthetics** (e.g., benzocaine, lidocaine, novacaine', Cetacaine')

-iacin: family of medications that fight *Staphylococcus*/"staph" and *Streptococcus*/ "strep" bacteria (e.g., erythromycin)

-itis: inflammation of

-oma: tumor (e.g., carcinoma, lymphoma)

-opsy: denotes a medical exam or inspection (e.g., biopsy)

-ostopy: implies a hole that is created surgically (e.g., tracheostopy)

-otomy/-ectomy: implies the surgical removal of something (e.g., tracheotomy, laryngectomy, tonsillectomy)

15.3 VOCABULARY

The following is a list of terms including bolded words from the text, as well as others we deem important additions to every singer's vocabulary. Some terms may be used in more ways than those listed here. For terms having more than one definition, only the definitions that support this text are included. Pronunciations are given in **phonetic symbols** and taken directly from the online Oxford Advanced Learner's Dictionary for terms that are often mispronounced. If you are uncertain about a pronunciation, you can use the audio option on the dictionary website: http://www.oxfordadvancedlearnersdictionary. com. When a pronunciation was unavailable, one was created by the author.

A

Abduct [æb'dʌkt]: the moving apart of the vocal folds into an open position.

Acetaminophen [ə͵siːtəˈmɪnəfen]: a common medication used to decrease pain and fever without decreasing inflammation. Found in tylenol® products.

Acquired: opposite of congenital. Developed after birth.

Acute [əˈkjuːt]: describes illnesses or symptoms that come on suddenly, need urgent attention, and last a short time.

Acute Nodules: a nodular-like thickening at the pmgc that appears with heavy hard performing and then recovers very quickly with voice rest, getting reabsorbed within a few days. Acute nodules that seem particular to opera singers.

Adduct [ˈædʌkt]: the drawing together of the vocal folds into a closed position. You can remember the difference between adduct and abduct by thinking of "*add*ing" the folds *together*.

Adenoids [ˈædənɔɪdz]: see **tonsils**.

Aditus [ˈædətəs]: an entrance or opening into a cavity such as the pharynx (aditus pharyngis) or larynx (aditus laryngis).

Adrenaline [əˈdrenəlɪn]: a hormone, also known as epinephrine, produced by your brain's medulla in its adrenal gland. Your brain triggers its adrenal gland to secrete adrenaline when it senses that you are frightened. The secreted adrenaline decreases your body's water flow, expands your lungs, increases your blood flow, and causes your heart to beat faster and more forcefully; all this prepares your muscles for a fight or flight. This adrenaline surge empowers your muscles to have a stronger contraction, but the surge also makes the contraction harder to achieve with the same stimulation. Singers who have experienced an adrenaline rush prior to performance describe a pounding heart, dry mouth and throat, shortness of breath, and difficulty singing a piece the way they practiced it.

Amplitude [ˈæmplɪtuːd]: the distance a vibrating object travels from the midline. We perceive amplitude as loudness and we measure amplitude in decibels. This distance is greatest when singing a high pitch loudly. However, singing a lower pitch at the same intensity/loudness would have the same amplitude.

Analgesics [ˌænəlˈdʒiːzɪk]: commonly known as pain killers, analgesics are over-the-counter or prescription medications that offer pain relief.

Anesthesia [ˌænəsˈθiːʒə]: literally "a state of decreased sensation or awareness." Topical anesthesia is achieved by applying an anesthetic (numbing substance) superficially, via spraying or rubbing, to numb a specific area. Local anesthesia is created by directly injecting an anesthetic into one specific point under the skin as given for a tooth cavity filling. Regional anesthesia is created by administering an anesthetic through injection or an iv to block the nerve supply to a large area of the body such as below the waist for a c-section baby delivery. General anesthesia is created through a combination of inhaled anesthetic gases and intravenous anesthetic medications (dripping one or more anesthetic medications into an iv to flow throughout the entire bloodstream) in order to cause amnesia and desensitize the whole body for invasive surgeries. General anesthesia is usually induced with an iv medication and then maintained with an anesthesia vapor that is a derivative of ether. Colloquially, we call general anesthesia "putting a patient to sleep," but this "sleep" involves an anesthetized brain that will not respond to pain or physical manipulations.

Note: Be mindful of undergoing regional anesthesia. Regional anesthesia numbs nerves, and although the numbness usually resolves within three to six months, a period of numbness can be a problem for any professional musician relying on his or her body to perform! Anesthesiologist Dr. Kenneth P. Gross advised a professional guitarist to actually undergo general anesthesia instead of regional anesthesia for an arm surgery. His patient refused and had to refrain from playing for three months until sensation returned in his arm.

Anesthesiologist, Dr. Kenneth P. Gross, e-mail message to author, January 7, 2011.

Anesthesiologist [ˌænəsˌθiːziˈɑːlədʒɪst]: an MD or DDS (dentist) who has completed four years of undergraduate education, four years of medical school, and four years of anesthesia residency (studying and administering anesthesia). The anesthesiologist may then choose to go on and do a cardiac, pediatric, pain management, or intensive care subspecialization. There is no laryngology subspecialty for anesthesiologists. The otolaryngologist has already specialized in anesthesia when he became a surgeon.

Anesthetics [ˌænəsˈθetɪks]: over-the-counter or prescription drugs used to numb or reduce sensation.

Angioedema [ˌændʒiouˈɪˈdiːmə]: an inflammatory reaction of blood vessel dilation similar to hives. Often brought on by angiotensin-converting enzyme inhibitors (aspirin, penicillin) or nonsteroidal anti-inflammatory agents found in medications such as "-cycline" and "-mycin" family antibiotics.

Anterior: Latin for "before." Toward the front.

Anterior Commissure [ˈkɑːmɪʃʊr]: the area toward the front of the neck where the vocal folds come together and meet just below and behind the thyroid notch.

Antitussive [ˌæntiˈtʌsɪv]: cough suppressant.

Aorta [eɪˈɔːrtə]: the biggest blood vessel in the body, stemming from the heart and branching off into the head, neck, arms, chest, abdomen, and legs. It is the body's main supplier of oxygenated blood.

Aperiodic [ˌeɪpɪriˈɑːdɪk]: irregular. In regard to the voice, aperiodic vibrations create an aperiodic sound. Vocal aperiodicity will sound complex, not clean and pure. Descriptions of aperiodic sounds include hoarseness, breathiness, unsteady pitch, diplophonia, or any combination of these.

Aphonia [eɪˈfouniə]: literally "no voice." Refers to the inability to produce any phonation.

Appoggio [aˈpadʒɔ]: from the italian verb *appoggiare*, which means "to lean." This term is used by classical singers when referring to leaning on the breath to support a sound. The "appoggio" or "lean" aptly describes the sensation felt by singers when striving to:

1. Maintain the contraction of the inhalation muscles (sensed by the diaphragm's pressure on the viscera and the expanded ribs)
2. Delay or slow the contraction of the exhalation muscles (i.e., the abdominal wall muscles, as well as those between the ribs)

While singing. This concentrated effort tries to delay the diaphragm's passive ascent on exhalation and keep air in the lungs for as long as possible. By maintaining or "leaning on" the tensions of inhalation while singing, the lungs are able to remain filled with air longer, exhalation is suspended, and subglottal pressure remains consistent.

Approximate [əˈprɑːksɪmeɪt]: draw together or bring near. When vocal folds approximate completely they are adducted. See **adduct.**

Aryepiglottic Folds [ˌeriˌepɪˈglɑːtɪk]: folds containing ligaments and muscle and covered with membranous tissue. They make up side portions of the aryepiglottic rim that encircles the laryngeal vestibule. When the muscles in the aryepiglottic folds contract, they have a sphincter-like effect on the laryngeal vestibule, narrowing the space inside the vestibule.

Aryepiglottic Sphincter [ˌeriepɪˈglɑːtɪk ˈsfɪŋktər]: describes the muscular attribute of the aryepiglottic rim of the laryngeal vestibule's outlining walls. The aryepiglottic folds tense with swallowing, creating a sphincter-like constriction to help keep food and liquids out of the airway. This action pulls the larynx away from the back wall of the pharynx, stretching open the esophageal entrance and allowing food to pass in two streams around the larynx and into the esophagus. Its contraction may also create a resonator (the laryngeal vestibule or **epilarynx**) within a resonator (the pharynx) and contribute to a vocal phenomenon many call the singer's formant. (See 14.3 How Are Opera Singers Heard over an Orchestra without Amplification?)

Arytenoids] [əˈrɪtənɔɪdz]: Greek for "ladle-like." Paired cartilages that sit like saddles on top of the cricoid cartilage. They can slide and rock, as well as pivot. These cartilages tend to be very pronounced and well defined in trained singers.

Aspirate [ˈæspəreɪt]: to inhale fluid into the lungs.

Aspirate Onset [ˈæspərət]: a breathy onset. Allowing breath to escape before a tone, as in "he."

Asthenic [esˈθenɪk]: weak, not strong.

Atrophy [ˈætrəfi]: the weakening or deterioration of a tissue (such as a muscle) or organ.

B

Bernoulli Effect [bərˈnuːli]: Daniel Bernoulli was a seventeenth-century Swiss scientist who discovered a principle of physics in which moving air or fluid has less density than stagnant air or fluid. In other words, as air or fluid travels through a narrowed space, it speeds up, and as the speed of the moving air or fluid increases, pressure decreases. This is known as the Bernoulli Effect and can be applied to explain phonation. As air passes between the narrowed space of the vocal folds it speeds up, decreasing pressure and drawing the vocal folds together. Air rebuilds under the vocal folds, blows them apart, then travels up between the folds with increasing speed, drawing the folds back together again. Each time the folds get drawn together and are blown apart makes up a cycle. Repetition of the cycles results in a vibratory pattern that we hear as phonation. The Bernoulli Effect also explains how a healthy, easy onset is produced as well.

Bilateral [ˌbaɪˈlætərəl]: relating to or occurring on both sides.

Board Certified: a term used to distinguish those physicians who have passed all requirements in a specialty field and have been tested and approved by a board of specialists in the specialty field. The certification grants them the privilege of practicing the specialty at a hospital.

Botulism [ˈbaːtʃəlɪzəm]: outpatient procedure of injecting botulinum toxin (commercially known as BOTOX®) to temporarily weaken nerve innervation to specific muscles. This toxin is especially helpful in counteracting the vocal spasms that accompany spasmodic dysphonia and can be injected every four to six months into the vocalis muscle to prevent hyperadduction or into the **posterior cricoarytenoid muscles** to prevent hyperabduction. It can also be injected, with less success, to diminish a wobble in the voice brought on by an essential tremor. The toxin may be administered directly into the vocal fold through the mouth or via a flexible scope placed in the nose. Most injections, however, are done by passing a needle into the skin on the front of the neck and passing through cricothyroid membrane using an EMG (electromyography) needle that records muscle activity to allow for precise placement. This toxin is also used cosmetically to reduce wrinkles. Singers should carefully consider the cosmetic use of BOTOX®. If done improperly, BOTOX® injections can temporarily paralyze muscles involved in facial expression. Additionally, injections around the mouth can cause temporary weakness of the lips and alter lip closure, similar to the effect of getting novocain from the dentist but lasting days, weeks, or even up to four months. Such weakness has the potential to change a person's annunciation of words.

BOTOX® ['boʊtɑːks]: see **botulism.**

Bowing ['boʊwɪŋ]: a condition in which the vocal folds adduct, but meet only at the top and bottom, making phonation difficult. Occurs when the thyroarytenoid muscles atrophy or are traumatized. Often happens with old age and is a symptom of presbylarynx.

Buccal Cavity ['bə-kəl]: see **oral cavity.**

C

Candida albicans: see oral *Candida.*

Capillary ['kæpəleri]: literally "hair-like." The tiniest member of the blood vessel family. About 0.0008 mm in diameter, they connect the smallest veins (**venules**) with the smallest arteries (**arterioles**). The larynx contains venules and capillaries only. No arteries, arterioles, or veins.

Carotid Arteries [kəˈrɑːtɪd ɑːrtəriz]: two significant blood vessels running along the front right and left sides of the neck. Both are branches supplied by the aorta and together the two supply most of the blood to the neck and head.

Cauterize ['kɔːtəraɪz]: to destroy tissue by applying heat. Accidentally burning yourself on the stove is cauterization. Cauterizing is useful in sealing off or removing tissue. A surgeon may cauterize (seal) blood vessels with the heat of a laser as he operates to prevent excess blood loss. He may also cauterize (remove) abnormal tissues that contain contagious disease. (See 10.14 Laryngeal Papilloma.) Electrocautery can be done with a bovie or chemical cautery can be done with silver nitrate.

Central: at or near the center. Opposite of peripheral.

Cetacaine® ['setəkeɪn]: a brand name for an anesthetic containing benzocaine that is sprayed into the nose to counteract the discomfort of nasendoscopies or into the mouth to numb the gag reflex occasionally triggered during oral endoscopies.

Chink: any narrow gap or opening. See **mutational chink** and **glottal gap.**

Chronic: opposite of acute. Describes illnesses or symptoms that persist indefinitely or longer than three months without change.

Cilia ['sɪliə]: tiniest hairs in the nostrils (not the ones visible) that sweep things into the sinuses. In this book, we also mention the hair-like *ciliated* cells in the ear and the areas of *ciliated* columnar respiratory epithelium that line the larynx.

Coloratura: originally from the German *Koloratur*, meaning an "elaborate ornamentation" of the melody. Describes an agile voice, usually female, that is able to sing consecutive ascending and descending pitches very quickly, as well as execute pitch leaps and *fioriture* (Italian "flourished" melodies, once called *canto figurato*).[1]

Concave: a surface that scoops inward, like a bowl. Opposite of **convex.**

Confidential Speech: well-pitched, abdominally supported speech that is no louder or softer than if speaking to someone an arm's length away. *If you can't touch them, you shouldn't be talking to them* is a helpful maxim.

---

[1] Coloratura is not originally from the Italian *colorare*, meaning "to color," and is not exclusive to high voices as often claimed. Richard Boldrey, *Guide to Operatic Roles & Arias* (Dallas: Pst...Inc., 1994), 12.

Congenital [kən'dʒenɪtl]: describes a trait or disorder you're born with, whether it be hereditary, influenced by pregnancy, or contracted in the birth canal.

Note: Be careful that you don't confuse congenital as being synonymous with genetic. Genetic describes only traits that are inherited, can be passed on to offspring, and are therefore present prior to birth. Congenital traits may or may not be inherited or present prior to birth. A congenital trait may be contracted in the birth canal, such as syphilis.

Contact Ulcer: a breakdown of laryngeal mucosa covering the arytenoids or the vocal fold epithelium covering the vocal process. Some believe it's a distinct disorder and some that it's an early-stage (immature) granuloma. Almost always occurs with reflux.

Convex ['kɑ:nveks]: a surface that curves outward, like an upside-down bowl. Opposite of concave.

Corniculates [kɔ:rn'nɪkjələts]: a pair of small horn-shaped projections of cartilage, one situated on top of each arytenoid. They don't develop until the teenage years.

Cover Wave: the motion of the true vocal folds' looser outer layers moving over the folds' denser inner layers during vocal fold vibration. The wave passes through the cover layers over and over again with fluidity, like ripples in a pond, closing the folds from front to back and bottom to top. Healthy cover waves are symmetrical and continuous. This term is coined in this book to replace the widely accepted but inaccurate term "mucosal wave" when referring to the motion of the true vocal folds.

Cranial ['kreɪniəl]: comes from the Latin word for skull, *cranium*. Having to do with the skull or head.

Cricoarytenoid Arthritis [ˌkraɪkoʊə'rɪtənɔɪd]: like any joints, the cricoarytenoid joints can get arthritis. Severe cases affecting arytenoid rotation may require a **tracheostomy**, because the arytenoids adduct the folds to protect the airway and abduct the folds for respiration.

Cricothyroid Muscles [ˌkraɪkoʊ'θaɪrɔɪd]: raise pitch on contraction by tilting the thyroid cartilage down in front, away from the signet portion of the cricoid, and thus lengthening the vocal folds. There are two sets: the oblique (lower horn) and the recta/straight (superior lower thyroid cartilage wall). The superior laryngeal nerve of the vagus innervates both sets.

Cuneiforms ['kju:nɪəfɔ:rmz]: Latin for "wedge form." Help keep the entrance to the larynx open by supporting and pulling taut the aryepiglottic folds. These tiny but crucial yellowish rods are **elastic cartilages** and don't develop until the teenage years.

Cycles Per Second: a measurement also described as **hertz**. For our purposes, this phrase refers to how many times the vocal folds complete a full period.

Cyst: a clogged mucous duct in the superficial lamina propria that causes a well-defined membranous sac to form. It rests on the vocal ligament and is often embedded in the fold's muscular layer. A cyst is firm and will usually irritate the opposite vocal fold during phonation and cause that fold to swell.

D

Decibel ['desɪbel]: an acoustical unit of measurement for relative sound intensity or loudness based on average human perception. Zero decibels is imperceptible to the human ear. One decibel equals the softest sound that can be detected by the average human ear.

Deglutition [diglu'tɪʃn]: swallowing. The mechanics of a swallow are as follows: 1. Tongue pushes food or liquid back. 2. Soft palate closes up against back wall of pharynx, closing nasopharynx. 3. The food bolus is pushed down into the vallecula, the pocket between the base of the tongue and the epiglottis. 4. The hyoid and larynx pull up and forward as the epiglottis folds over the vocal folds. 5. The food bolus flows in two streams around the larynx and down into the esophagus.

Depressors: muscles that lower the larynx with contraction. They are paired with **elevators** that relax as depressors contract.

Deviated Nasal Septum: a crooked line down the midline of the nose where there should be a straight one. The **nasal septum** may be abnormal due to a broken nose bone, but most often it is due to a fault in the cartilage or a break where the bone and cartilage fuse. See **nasal septum.**

Diaphragm [ˈdaɪəfræm]: an unpaired muscle shaped like an upside-down, double-domed salad bowl that attaches along the bottom ribs and separates the abdomen from the thorax. The diaphragm contracts upon inspiration, lowering, and drawing the lungs down with it to expand them vertically, assisting them as they fill with air. It relaxes with expiration, returning to its higher resting position. Because its contraction helps inspiration only, it is an inhalatory muscle.

Diaphragmatic Displacement [daɪəfrəˈmætɪk]: any amount of diaphragm contraction. When the diaphragm contracts, it lowers, leaving its resting position. In other words, it is displaced. Diaphragmatic displacement occurs as the lungs fill with air, and not as the lungs expel air. The diaphragm simply returns to its resting position with exhalation.

Diplophonia [ˌdɪpləˈfoʊniə]: literally "double phonation." Caused when two separate sources vibrate simultaneously. If you hear what sounds like two different pitches simultaneously coming out of your mouth while you talk or sing, you're not crazy! This phenomenon often occurs with unilateral lesions. Diplophonia may also occur when extreme muscle tension pulls the false vocal folds together so that they vibrate above the true vocal folds.

Disorders: abnormal conditions.

Dissection: involves cutting a structure in its original state in order to holistically understand the relationship between its internal components, as well as its relationship to all of its surrounding structures.

Dysarthria [dɪsˈɑːrθriə]: most often refers to poor articulation (slurred speech) due to tongue or laryngeal muscle impairment brought on by nerve damage. Some medications can also cause temporary dysarthria.

Dysphonia [dɪsˈfoʊniə]: abnormal voice such as hoarseness.

E

Edema [ɪˈdiːmə]: adj. Edematous [ɪˈdemətəs]. Commonly called swelling. An abnormal accumulation of excessive serous fluid (a.k.a. thin, protein-bound water) outside the blood vessels and in the lining of any injured or inflamed tissue.

Elastic Cartilage: tissue that doesn't **ossify** but continues to stay flexible. Elastic cartilages of the larynx include the epiglottis, the superior portion of the arytenoid from the vocal process (allowing flexibility during abduction and adduction) up to the arytenoid apex, and the **corniculates,** which sit on top.[2]

Elastic Recoil: the spring-like return of soft tissue or muscle after excursion (moving away from its resting position). Your rib muscles begin to recoil after contracting to open the ribcage for an intake of breath. They want to return to their resting position, which helps create exhalation.

Electroglottogram [ɪˌlektroʊˈglɑːtəgræm]: also called an EGG. A device that measures vocal fold contact via electrodes attached to the outside of the neck at the thyroid cartilage. The electrodes pick up an electrical current made when your folds come into contact with each vibration.

Elevators: muscles that raise the larynx with contraction. They are paired with **depressors** that relax as elevators contract.

Emesis [ˈeməsɪs]: vomiting or throwing up.

Endarterectomy [ˌendartəˈrektəmi]: an operation to clean plaque buildup from an artery to restore blood flow.

Endocrine [ˈendəkrɪn]: internal secretions that are carried and distributed by the bloodstream, such as hormones.

Endoscope: a lighted instrument specifically designed to be inserted into a natural opening on the body and allow visual examination of an internal area. Many types offer magnification as well. The laryngoscope is a type of endoscope. (See **laryngoscope**.) This book discusses several types of laryngoscopes: the rigid oral endoscope, the flexible nasendoscope, the operating laryngoscope, and the intubating laryngoscope. To perform an upper gastrointestinal endoscopy, an extra-long flexible endoscope is used.

Endotracheal Tube [ˌendoʊˈtreɪkiəl]: also called an ETT, the tube placed in the trachea and used to ventilate a patient during surgery.

Epiglottis [ˌepɪˈglɑːtɪsa]: a thin, leaf-shaped cartilage of the larynx that projects up behind and slightly below the tongue and covers the airway during swallowing.

Epilarynx [ˌepɪˈlærɪŋks]: see **laryngeal vestibule**.

Epithelium [ˌepɪˈθiliəm]: tissue that forms the most superficial cover on various internal and external body surfaces. Most epithelium emits some kind of secretion such as mucus or sweat. Epidermis (skin) and the superficial layer of the true vocal folds are types of epithelium. Epithelium often makes up the superficial layer of mucosa as well.

Erythema [ˌerəˈθimə]: redness due to inflammation.

Esophageal Sphincter [iˈsɑːfədʒiːl ˈsfɪŋktər]: a valve-like opening that lets food into the stomach after swallowing and keeps food in the stomach during digestion. The esophagus has two sphincters—an upper and a lower.

Note: Eww! To fully understand what a sphincter is, think of your bum. Your esophageal sphincter looks identical to the sphincter of your bum. So, when you burp, it's not unlike flatulence. The two release different odors due to emissions coming from places dealing with differing stages of digestion.

Esophagus [iˈsɑːfəgəs]: also known as the gullet, this approximately 10-inch-long food tube extends from just behind the larynx and posterior to the arytenoids, down through an opening in the diaphragm and into the stomach. When you swallow, the larynx rises slightly and tips forward. As a result and with a little help from the thyroepiglottic muscles, the

---

2 K. Sato et al., "Distribution of Elastic Cartilage in the Arytenoids and Its Physiologic Significance," *Annals of Otology, Rhinology, and Laryngology* 99, no. 5 Pt 1 (May 1990): 363.

epiglottis folds over, protecting the entrance to the trachea, while the pocket-like entrance to the esophageal sphincter is stretched open to receive what you're swallowing. Unless you are talking while you're eating, this reflex is involuntary and won't get mixed up! Nothing that is swallowed will actually touch the vocal folds but will travel around the larynx in two streams and deposit directly into the esophagus. The presence of liquid or a food bolus triggers this tube of smooth muscle to involuntarily squeeze everything toward the stomach in wave-like motions called peristalsis.

Essential Tremor: a neurological disorder causing trembling of a body part. Essential means not associated with other diseases. An essential tremor begins gradually, usually affecting the hands first, then eventually the head and voice and worsens with caffeine, stress, lack of sleep, and exposure to extreme temperatures. Its etiology is unknown but seems to be genetic or brought on by old age.

Etiology [ˌiːtiˈɑːlədʒi]: the cause or root of something, such as any given pathology.

Expectorant [ɪkˈspektərənt]: a medication that assists in bringing mucus up from the lungs. An example is guaifenesin.

F

Fach [fɑːkh]: German for "type," as in type of operatic singing voice. The German Fach System categorizes operatic voices based on their size, color, tessitura, and range. An opera singer who has determined her Fach can pursue a longer, healthier career by only agreeing to perform roles that match her Fach. The Fach label also helps the person casting a show to assign roles successfully. Take a role in Mozart's *Marriage of Figaro,* for example. Due to light orchestral accompaniment (determines voice size), the highest and lowest sung pitches (determines voice range), the most commonly sung pitches (determines tessitura), and the youthful nature of her character (determines color), Susanna is most successfully sung by a light lyric soprano and not by a dramatic soprano or spinto, who may strain in efforts not to be too loud or sound too powerful to be a young newlywed.

Flexible Fiberoptic Nasendoscope: instrument used to view the larynx via the nose. The long skinny tube contains a bundle of five light strands that illuminate the larynx for viewing and recording purposes. See **nasendoscopy.**

Formalin [ˈfɔːrmələn]: a disinfectant and germicide solution of water, formaldehyde, and usually a small amount of methanol used to preserve biopsied tissue sent for microscopic examination at the lab.

Free Margin: see **medial edges.**

Frequency: the frequency is the objective measurement of the vocal folds', or any sound-generating device's, periodic (meaning healthy, consistent, regular) vibrating rate. Frequency equals the number of times per second that the vocal folds complete a cycle of vibration.

Fundamental Frequency: the rate at which a waveform repeats per unit of time.[3] When used in a vocal context, this translates to the number of times the vocal folds vibrate per second. Any vibrating source with regular/periodic vibrations has a fundamental frequency.

G

Gastroesophageal Reflux Disease [ˌgæstrəiˌsɑːfəˈdʒiːl]: a chronic condition in which stomach contents spill into the esophagus due to acidic irritation, overeating, weak motility action (ability to push acid back into the stomach), or a weak lower esophageal sphincter. Singers often develop GERD by eating a lot after a late performance and going to bed shortly thereafter. GERD is also common in singers due to the vigorous diaphragmatic and abdominal action used in Western classical singing that jostles stomach contents and triggers burping. (See 5.10 Reflux and Heartburn and **laryngopharyngeal reflux**.)

General Anesthesia: see **anesthesia** and **intubation** and General Anesthesia and Intubation in 12.1 (Aspects of the Surgical Process that Concern Singers).

Glottal Fry: also called vocal fry, creak voice, or pulse register. Glottal fry is considered the lowest register of any given human voice. However, rather than a series of pitches produced in a similar manner like a true vocal register is, glottal fry is noise and has no perceptible pitch. Glottal fry consists of vocal fold vibrations that are aperiodic and vary from 20 to 50 cycles per second. Frequency is impossible to track and precise pitches are impossible to detect. As a result, we can safely say glottal fry is pitchless. In actuality, because of our ears' limitations, we are likely to perceive any sung pitch below 70 Hz as glottal fry![4]

Glottal Gap: also called a glottal **chink**. A general term for any opening in the vocal folds' closure. Glottal gaps may be considered normal or pathological. Bowed vocal folds involve a glottal gap that is not considered normal. A lesion such as a cyst or polyp commonly prevents the folds from closing completely, and air leaks through the glottal gaps above and below the lesion during phonation. A *posterior* glottal gap is a triangular gap left between the vocal fold processes (the cartilaginous portion of the folds) during adduction. The interarytenoideus muscles must be able to contract to close this gap in order to complete adduction. A posterior glottal gap may be considered pathological if a lot of interarytenoid swelling or pachyderma prevents complete closure. A mutational chink is a particular type of posterior glottal gap that is generally not considered pathological. A mutational chink is normally observed in healthy preadult vocal folds (especially females) and is associated with interarytenoideus weakness.

Glottal Onset: beginning vowel phonation with the false and true folds closed and blowing them apart as in "uh oh." Its articulation quality is similar to a consonant, and when used habitually in a hard, tense way, it can be vocally tiring.

Glottis: the space from the anterior commissure to the vocal process ends of the arytenoids.

Granuloma [ˌɡrænjəˈloʊmə]: literally "grainy tumor." Redundant tissue buildup from chronic irritation or infection. Often occurs in the posterior larynx with reflux or in the anterior larynx from intubation trauma. A unilateral lesion can cause granuloma to form on the opposite fold. Usually takes eight weeks of voice therapy, hydration, and rest to heal.

Guaifenesin: an expectorant that thins mucus and encourages the production of plentiful thin mucus to lubricate inflamed trachea and bronchi and make it easier to cough up from the lungs.

[3] Ronald J. Baken and Robert F. Orlikoff, *Clinical Measurement of Speech and Voice* (San Diego: Singular, 2000), 147.

[4] "Chapter 10 Vocal Registers," *Tutorial based on Ingo Titze's Principles of Voice Production* (Englewood Cliffs, NJ: Prentice Hall, 1994). The National Center for Voice and Speech, http://www.ncvs.org/ncvs/tutorials/voiceprod/tutorial/voluntary.html, accessed August 21, 2011.

H

Hemorrhage ['heməridʒ]: a burst/ruptured blood vessel. Hemorrhage is also used as a verb to describe active blood loss.

Hertz [hɜːrts]: abbreviation Hz. A unit of frequency measurement equaling 1 cycle/second.

Hirano ['hirənoʊ]: Miranu Hirano, MD, PhD, born in Japan, 1935.

Histology: cellular or microscopic make-up of any given tissue.

Hoarseness: also called dysphonia. A harsh, noisy voice quality that occurs when there is a disruption in the periodicity of vocal fold vibrations or oscillations. Any disruption in the vocal folds' phonatory pattern allows air to escape and results in a hoarse sound. Such disruptions include anything from minor edema to serious pathologies and often stem from vocal abuse or misuse. Neurological disorders such as paralysis can cause hoarseness as well.

Hyaline ['haɪələn]: translucent.

Hyaline Cartilage ['haɪələn]: fibrous tissue that ossifies with age. Hyaline cartilages in the larynx (i.e., the thyroid, cricoid, and most of the arytenoid) begin to ossify from the top down in the late twenties.

Hyoid ['haɪɔɪd]: literally Greek for "u-shaped." Refers to the horseshoe-shaped bone originating at the base of the tongue.

Hypertrophy [haɪˈpɜːrtrəfi]: the enlargement of an organ or tissue due to an increase in size, not number, of the organ's or tissue's cells.

Hyponatremia [ˌhaɪpoʊnəˈtrimiə]: also known as water intoxication. Occurs when the body's sodium levels are too low. This rare imbalance is more commonly found in athletes who drink a lot of water after sweating intensely but fail to replenish the lost salt. Too little sodium in the body causes tissues to swell, including those in the brain, which can lead to intoxicated behavior, seizures, coma, or even death. Depending on performance demands and physique, the average singer's body needs around three quarts/twelve cups/seventy-two ounces of water each day. (About 20% of this amount will come from the food we eat.) The average kidneys, however, are capable of processing around sixteen quarts each day! So the danger of becoming hyponatremic is unlikely and lies more in how fast you drink water and not so much in the amount of water you take in. Even drinking a lot of water very quickly is unlikely to trigger hyponatremia, because the body will often protect itself by spontaneously vomiting whatever it cannot handle.

Note: Did you know you can count your swallows to keep track of water intake? Eight swallows of water roughly equals eight ounces or one cup.

Hyperthyroidism: also called hyperthyroid disorder. Overactive thyroid disorder in which the thyroid gland (different from the thyroid cartilage) is inflamed and makes too much thyroid hormone. The change in hormone levels can cause swelling in the superficial lamina propria, resulting in a deepening of the voice. The front of the neck may be sore to touch. The condition can also cause general fatigue, general muscle weakness (including pharyngeal, facial, or laryngeal muscles and resulting in possible vocal fatigue, breathiness, or hoarseness), nervousness, irritability, increased perspiration, and weight loss. Surgery may correct a hyperthyroid but can put the RLN and SLN nerves that innervate the larynx at risk of damage. (See Nerve Damage in 12.1 Aspects of the Surgical Process that Concern Singers.)

Hypothyroidism: also called hypothyroid disorder. Underactive thyroid gland disorder in which the thyroid gland (different from the cartilage) is inflamed and doesn't make enough thyroid hormone to regulate your metabolism. The change in hormone levels can cause swelling in the superficial lamina propria, resulting in a deepening of the voice. The front of the neck may be sore to touch. The condition can also cause general fatigue, general muscle weakness (including pharyngeal, facial, and laryngeal muscles and resulting in possible vocal fatigue, breathiness, or hoarseness), weight gain, muscle cramps, depression, and irritability.

I

Iatrogenic [aɪˌætrəˈdʒenɪk]: an adverse effect caused inadvertently by a medical professional while administering medical care.

Idiopathic [ˌɪdiəˈpɑːθək]: having unknown cause.

In Phase: vibrating symmetrically, producing a periodic tone. The opposite of "**out of phase**."

Indirect Laryngoscopy [ˈlærɪŋgɑːskəpi]: also called mirror imaging. Using a mirror inserted into the oral cavity to observe the vocal folds. (See The Mirror in 8.3 Instruments Used in the Clinic.)

Inferior: an anatomical reference term for under or lower in relation to another reference point.

Innervation: the stimulation of a body part via nerves.

Intensity: the degree of loudness or volume.

Interarytenoideus Muscles [ɪntɜːrəˈrɪtənɔɪdiəs]: also referred to as the arytenoideus muscles. Made up of the paired oblique arytenoid muscles and the unpaired transverse arytenoid muscle. This set of two muscles connects the arytenoids and is innervated by the RLN, contracting to bring the arytenoids closer together. It helps to complete vocal fold closure on adduction by closing the cartilaginous portion of the vocal folds (area 7 to 9).

Interarytenoid Space [ˌɪntɜːrəˈrɪtənɔɪd]: the area of the larynx between the arytenoid cartilages.

Intermediate: an anatomical reference term for lying between two points.

Intubation: the proper name used to describe the process of placing the endotracheal tube in the trachea.

J

Jitter: refers to slight differences between one cycle of vibration and another. In other words, jitter is a variation in the fundamental frequency or pitch of the voice. While these small variations do alter the fundamental pitch, they do not *audibly* hinder the sound quality of the voice.

K

Keratinized Tissue [ˈkerətɪnaɪzd]: tough "cornified" tissue, such as a fingernail or callus, that protects from abrasion. A newly formed vocal fold polyp is soft and often fluid filled but can keratinize after rubbing against the opposite fold during phonation.

L

Lamina Propria [ˈlæmɪnə ˈprouprɪə]: a thin connective tissue that lies under the epithelium with three layers of different consistencies. The superficial lamina propria can be considered a gel-like

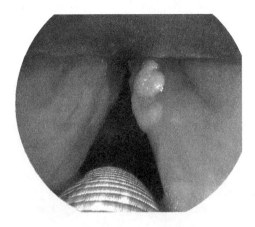

Figure 15.3a Laryngeal Carcinoma
Photo of cancerous growth on the right vocal fold taken through operating laryngoscope just prior to surgical removal.

pillow for the folds, and the intermediate lamina propria (tissue like soft rubberbands) and deep lamina propria (tissue like strands of cotton) make up the vocal ligament.

Laparotomy [ˌlæpəˈrɑːtəmi]: a surgical incision in the abdominal wall in order to access the abdominal cavity.

Laryngeal [ləˈrɪndʒiəl]: of or pertaining to the larynx.

Laryngeal Carcinoma [ləˈrɪndʒiəl ˌkɑːrsɪˈnoʊmə]: full name, laryngeal squamous cell carcinoma. Carcinoma is the generic term for cancerous growth (malignant changes) originating in the membranes (skin or tissues) that line the body's organs. Carcinomic growth is usually identified by its white, cottage cheese–like lesions. One example is squamous cell carcinoma, which begins in mucosa. It is one of the most common skin cancers and the most common form of lung and laryngeal cancer. Laryngeal squamous cell carcinoma generally stems from smoking and/or alcoholism. It often causes hoarseness. Other symptoms may include bad breath (a specific smell unique to cancer), sore throat, persistent cough, referred "earache," and lump in the neck. (See Figure 15.3a.)

Laryngeal Saccule [ləˈrɪndʒiəl ˈsækjul]: a membranous sac or pocket containing mucus-secreting glands that superficially hydrate the true folds below it. It is situated between the false folds and the inside surface of the thyroid wall, just above the true folds.

Laryngeal Web [ləˈrɪndʒiəl]: scar tissue bond of laryngeal tissues formed anteriorly between the vocal folds, partially closing off the airway, and causing a voice to sound high, thin, and strained.

Laryngeal Vestibule: also called **epilarynx.** The whole area between the epiglottis and the true vocal folds. The rim of the laryngeal vestibule is called the aryepiglottic rim or, because it has muscular properties that allow it to narrow the vestibule like a sphincter, it may be called the aryepiglottic sphincter. See **aryepiglottic sphincter.**

Laryngectomy [ˌlærɪnˈdʒɛktəmi]: total or partial removal of the larynx. Often necessitated by laryngeal cancer or severe trauma to the larynx. Usually mandates a **tracheostomy** because without the larynx, the trachea is left unprotected. Alternative voice methods are resorted to such as the artificial larynx or esophageal speech.

Laryngitis [ˌlærɪnˈdʒaɪtɪs]: a general term for inflammation of the larynx. Laryngitis can result from irritation, infection, vocal misuse, or vocal overuse. Hoarseness and complete loss of voice are common symptoms of laryngitis.

Laryngologist [ˌlærɪŋˈgɑːlədʒɪst]: an otolaryngologist who specializes in disorders of the larynx and voice.

Laryngology [ˌlærɪŋˈgɑːlədʒi]: study of the larynx and its pathologies.

Laryngopharyngeal Reflux [læˌrɪŋgəˌfærɪnˈdʒiəl]: may or may not be a chronic condition (i.e., a type of GERD) in which stomach acid gets sloshed all the way up into the larynx and pharynx due to acidic irritation, overeating, or weak lower esophageal sphincter. Singers often trigger LPR by eating a lot after a late performance and going to bed shortly thereafter. LPR is also common in singers due to the vigorous diaphragmatic action used in Western classical singing that jostles stomach contents and triggers burping. LPR is a more serious type of GERD for singers, because the acid burns the tissues surrounding the vocal folds, making them swell and function less efficiently. (See **gastroesophageal reflux disease** and 5.10 Reflux and Heartburn.)

Laryngopharynx [læˌrɪŋgəˈfærɪŋks]: also called hypopharynx. The lower pharyngeal area beginning at the level of the hyoid bone and ending at the vocal folds and esophagus.

Laryngoplasty [læˌrɪŋgəˈplæsti]: general term referring to any surgery on the framework of the larynx. May or may not be a phonosurgery. Not microlaryngeal surgery.

Laryngoscope [læˈrɪŋgəskoʊp]: any endoscope designed to obtain a direct view of the larynx. There are three major laryngoscope categories discussed in this text: the clinical laryngoscopes, the operating laryngoscopes, and the intubating laryngoscopes. Those used in the clinic for diagnostic and recording purposes are equipped with a light, magnifying lens, and camera. They may be rigid or flexible, and of those two types, there are many brands and styles. An operating laryngoscope is a hollow metal tube that is inserted into a patient's mouth and down the pharynx, providing a noninvasive (i.e., no cutting involved) channel through which the surgeon can operate on the larynx. A light is inserted alongside the scope to illuminate the laryngeal vestibule. These come in a variety of shapes to offer slightly different laryngeal views and to suit different-sized necks. The surgeon's preference will depend on the type of microlaryngeal surgery being performed. Intubation laryngoscopes are thin, slightly curved, and commonly rigid instruments shaped similarly to a shoe horn. Once inserted, they provide a track to the larynx that guides the insertion of the endotracheal tube.

Laryngoscopy [lærɪŋˈgɑːskəpi]: generally refers to an outpatient procedure in which a clinician views the larynx in motion with one of two types of scopes: a rigid oral endoscope or a flexible nasendoscope. (See exception below.) When the exam is recorded on video, it's called a video laryngoscopy. When the exam involves strobe light illumination, it's referred to as laryngeal stroboscopy or strobolaryngoscopy. When recorded, it's a VLS. (See **video laryngeal stroboscopy** and 8.3 Instruments Used in the Clinic.) You may hear laryngoscopies categorized as macro- or microlaryngoscopies. "Macrolaryngoscopy" refers specifically to an exam that looks broadly and thoroughly at the larynx and entire vocal tract (as is done during a nasendoscopy). "Microlaryngoscopy" is used almost exclusively to refer to the exam of the vocal folds' free edges through an operating laryngoscope in the operating room. See **laryngoscope**.

Laryngospasm [læˈrɪŋgəspæzm]: a sudden contraction of the vocal folds and epiglottis to block the airway, as opposed to a pharyngeal reflex (a.k.a. "gag"), which causes the soft palate to rise.

Larynx ['lærɪŋks]: literally "throat" in Greek. A cartilaginous structure otherwise known as voice box that houses the vocal folds and protects the airway. Its development occurs as cartilage grows. The angle of the "Adam's Apple" protrusion in the male larynx is 90 degrees (from left to right) and is reached after pubescent growth spurt with a sudden laryngeal tilt alteration. The female's laryngeal growth is gradual and her thyroid prominence eventually reaches 120 degrees.

Lateral: from Latin term *latus*, meaning "side." An anatomical reference term for alongside of, a point away from the midline.

Lateral Excursion: the distance a fold travels away from the middle of the glottis during vibration.

Lesion ['liːʒn]: a specific area of abnormally altered tissue due to injury or disease.

Leukoplakia [luːkplkiə]: white patches of precancerous mucosal tumors that usually extend subepithelially and develop from constant irritation such as smoking and GERD. They must be watched carefully, as they can become malignant. (See Figures 15.3b and 15.3c.)

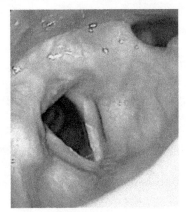

Figure 15.3b Leukoplakia
Whitish precancerous thickening of vocal fold cover presenting along the right vocal fold's medial edge 3 to 4 and affecting the left vocal fold's medial edge and superior surface 2 to 6.

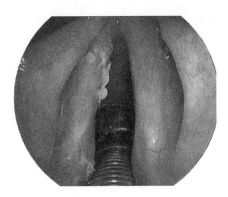

Figure 15.3c Possible Leukoplakia
White precancerous thickening of left vocal fold cover. Photo taken just prior to surgical removal.

Ligament: a band of strong connective tissue attaching cartilage to cartilage, bone to bone, or bone to cartilage.

Local Anesthesia: see **anesthesia**.

Lower Esophageal Sphincter [iˈsɑːfədʒiəl ˈsfɪŋktər]: the valve connecting the stomach and esophagus. See **esophageal sphincter**.

Lubricant: a substance that makes a surface slippery and decreases friction when another surface moves against it.

Lubricate: to make slippery.

Lymphatic Fluid [lɪmˈfætɪk]: a transparent yellowish watery serum that leaves the bloodstream to enter the body's vein-like lymphatic channels in order to carry cells and substances that fight infection and injury and begin the healing process.

M

Meatus [miˈeɪtəs]: "meatus" is both singular and plural. A passage or opening as in the upper, middle, and lower nasal meatus between the turbinates. A nasendoscope is passed through a meatus to obtain a view of the vocal folds.

Medial: toward the middle/midline.

Medial edge: the free vibrating portion of each true vocal fold.

Medialize [ˌmidiəlaɪˈz]: to come closer to the middle.

Membrane: thin, pliable tissue that connects structures, separate spaces, and organs and lines cavities.

Meniscus [məˈnɪskəs]: a "c"-shaped cartilage that acts as a cushion, partly separating a joint.

Methylxanthines [ˌmeθəlˈzænθiːn]: agents that are diuretics, smooth muscle relaxants, cardiac muscle stimulants, and central nervous system stimulants. Three are naturally present in foods: theobromine (in cocoa beans, tea, açaí berries, some sodas), theophylline (in teas, cocoa beans), and caffeine (in cocoa beans, teas, coffee).

Microdebrider [ˌmaɪkroʊdeˈbridər]: a long, thin, hollow surgical vacuum with a tiny blade rotating just inside one end. The electrical instrument is operated by a foot pedal and is designed to cut up extra tissue while suctioning it out of the airway.

Microlaryngeal Surgery [ˌmaɪkroʊləˈrɪndʒiəl]: also called laryngeal microsurgery. A surgery in which a microscope and small instruments are used to remove pathology from the larynx. All microlaryngeal vocal fold surgeries are phonosurgeries.

Mirror Imaging: see **indirect laryngoscopy** and The Mirror in 8.3 Instruments Used in the Clinic.

Mucolytic [ˌmjukəˈlɪtək]: a pharmaceutical agent that breaks down and hydrolyzes mucus to make it thinner.

Mucosa [mjuːˈkoʊzə]: also called **mucous membrane**. Nonkeratinizing moist epithelium made up of protein-bound water (glycoprotein). Mucosa lines body cavities that are involved in absorption and secretion such as the mouth, nose, inside of the lips, pharynx, most of the larynx, false vocal folds, trachea, lungs, urogenital tract, reproductive organs, esophagus, and gastrointestinal (GI) tract.

Mucosal Wave [mjuːˈkoʊzəl]: a term traditionally used to describe the vibratory motion of the cover over the body of the true vocal folds. Because the wave doesn't pass through the entire mucosa, however, calling the wave "mucosal" is technically incorrect. "Mucosal wave" may accurately be used to describe the pattern of vibration that occasionally will develop in the mucosa of the false folds with consistently practiced false fold phonation. See **cover wave**.

Mucous Membrane [ˈmjuːkəs]: see **mucosa**.

Mucus [ˈmjuːkəs]: adj. mucous. A clear fluid secreted by mucous membranes/mucosa to lubricate and protect. Ample, thin mucus denotes hydration. Thicker mucus is produced when the body is trying to digest certain foods or trying to protect itself and in some cases can be a sign of infection or dehydration. The slang for mucus secreted in the mouth is *spit*.

Muscle Tension Dysphonia [dɪsˈfoʊniə]: also called hyperkinetic vocal function. A voice disorder due to abnormal or severe muscle tension in the larynx. May develop out of compensation for an existing vocal fold lesion or simply from psychological stress.

Muscular Antagonism: for one skeletal muscle to contract, another must relax. All skeletal muscles except the diaphragm and the transverse arytenoid (a muscle of the interarytenoideus) are paired muscles, each with a muscular antagonist (e.g., the biceps and triceps muscles are paired; they have an antagonistic relationship). See **interarytenoideus**.

Mutational Chink: a specific type of posterior glottal gap that is an anatomical phenomenon seen in young (preadult) vocal folds, especially females, and contributes to a breathy sound. A mutational chink suggests a weak interarytenoideus muscle. They usually shrink with age or even earlier as good vocal technique is pursued and high range develops. Some women never get 100% closure. If a mutational chink continues to be present later in a woman's life, it is simply referred to as a posterior glottal gap and is not necessarily pathological. A woman who prefers using a breathier sound may never reach complete closure but still be considered by voice clinicians to have a normal and healthy voice. The bigger the gap is, the bigger the indication that something may be a problem. In singers, a bigger gap tends to be a concern, not only because breathiness limits vocal range and dynamics and is generally undesirable in most schools of singing, but also because less length of the fold is meeting for vibration, placing more stress on the anterior portion of the folds.

Myasthenia Laryngis [ˌmaɪjəsˈθiniə ləˈrɪndʒɪs]: also called bowed vocal folds. Vocal folds worn with overuse and plagued with dysphonia characterized by difficulty getting loud enough to be heard.

Myxedema [ˌmɪkxɪˈdiːmə]: severe hypothyroid disorder causing severe dryness and swelling.

N

Nares: nostrils or openings in the nose lined with hair.

Nasal Cavities: two passageways opening at the nose at one end and into the nasopharynx at the other. The passageways are separated by the nasal septum. Each passage is lined with ciliated epithelium and produces highly vascular mucus that catches and traps dust and **pathogens**. Air that passes through the nasal cavities is warmed, moistened, and filtered.

Nasal Septum [ˈseptəm]: cartilaginous midline in the nasal cavity that transforms to bone higher up in the nose.

Nasendoscopy [ˌneɪzenˈdɑːskəpi]: a video laryngoscopy exam that is done by passing a flexible wire containing a camera through the most open of three nasal passageways or meatus. Nasendoscopy views are not as close as with oral endoscopy, but going through the nose works better for children who don't sit still and patients with a sensitive gag reflex. Nasendoscopies are also necessary to diagnose vcd because the patient's normal talking and breathing can be better observed. A closer picture may be obtained by having the patient not swallow or cough for ten seconds while the camera is lowered into the aryepiglottic sphincter. A patient who does cough or swallow during this procedure will likely pass out due to the obstructed airway. (See 8.3 Instruments Used in the Clinic.)

Nasopharynx [ˌneɪzoʊˈfærɪŋks]: also called postnasal space. The area of the pharynx above the soft palate.

Nodules [ˈnɑːdʒuːlz]: literally "knots or calluses." Common pathology in preachers, teachers, lawyers, singers. Nodules can be either edematous or fibrous. Bilateral and callus-like in nature, nodules occur at the pmgc. See **point of maximum glottal contact**.

Noise: when any given vibration/vibratory cycle is aperiodic or irregular, noise is the result.

Nonkeratinizing Stratified Squamous cell epithelium [nɑːn ˈkerətɪnaɪzd ˈstrætɪfaɪd ˈskweɪməs ˌepɪˈθiliəm]: special tissue covering wet areas of the body that undergo wear and tear such as the mouth, esophagus, vagina, anal cavity, vocal folds, and parts of the larynx. Nonkeratinizing means the outer cell layer will not morph into a nonliving, tough protein substance (found in the outermost layer of skin [epidermis], as well as in hair and nails). Stratified squamous cell epithelium specifies a type of tissue made up of flat epithelial cells (such as the anterior surface of the epiglottis and the top rim of the aryepiglottic folds). The true vocal folds are covered by nonkeratinizing stratified squamous cell epithelium. Also call *nonkeratinized* stratified squamous cell epithelium. See **stratified squamous epithelium**.

O

Odynophagia [ˌoʊdɪnəˈfeɪʒə]: painful swallowing.

Odynophonia [ˌoʊdɪnəˈfoʊniə]: painful phonation.

Onset: see **vocal onset**.

Oral *Candida* [ˈkændɪdə]: the most common oral/laryngeal yeast infection, also known as thrush. Oral *Candida* is contagious fungus in the mouth characterized by a cottage cheese appearance and burning and implies immune system deficiency (often triggered from antibiotics). *Candida* lives in 10% of all people, but it is an opportunistic infection, meaning it won't develop on its own but rather has to have an opportunity to grow. It won't reveal itself unless some aspect of its environment changes, whether due to dryness, killed good bacteria, or steroids, for example. (See Figure 15.3d.)

Oral Cavity: also called the **buccal cavity** or *albicans*. Denotes the inner mucosa–lined mouth area, not surrounding outer skin.

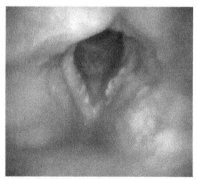

Figure 15.3d Oral *Candida*
Bilateral white fungal growth along the entire length of the right fold and areas 1 to 7 of the left fold.

Oral Endoscopy [ˈɔːrəl enˈdɑːskəpi]: the type laryngoscopy procedure that is done with a scope that goes in the mouth and is balanced right under the uvula, to look over and behind the tongue. Some patients have a hyper gag reflex and do not tolerate this well. The angle of the camera is 70 degrees, although there are 90-degree scopes that require full insertion to the back wall of the pharynx to get a full picture. The oral endoscopy distorts singing quality due to unnatural position of articulators and prohibits breathing through the nose. (See 8.3 Instruments Used in the Clinic.)

Oropharynx [ˌɔːroʊˈfærɪŋks]: the middle portion of the pharynx encompassing the space above the epiglottis and below the soft palate.

Osmolality [ˌɑːzməˈlɑːləti]: the number or concentration of compounds dissolved within a solution.

Ossify [ˈɑːsɪfaɪ]: harden. Due to their unique cellular makeup, **hyaline cartilages** in our bodies turn to bone (ossify) as we age. The process leading to ossification is called calcification, meaning the tissue has begun to develop hard calcium deposits and as a result loses pliability.

Ostium [ˈɑːstiəm]: small hole, mouth, opening, or **stoma** of something.

Otolaryngologist [ˌoʊtoʊlærɪŋˈgɑːlədʒist]: also called otorhinolaryngologist. A certified specialist in ear, nose, and throat disorders.

Otolaryngology [ˌoʊtoʊlærɪŋˈgɑːlədʒi]: a surgical specialization that follows becoming an md. The full name of this specialty is **otolaryngology-head and neck surgery**. Practitioners are called **otolaryngologists-head and neck surgeons**, specifically **otorhinolaryngologists** (ORL), and among laymen, **ENTs** (**ear, nose, and throat doctors**).

Otology [oʊˈtɑːlədʒi]: study of the ear and its pathologies.

Out of phase: asymmetric vocal fold vibrations, which produce all different frequencies and result in an aperiodic tone. The opposite of "**in phase**."

P

Pachyderma [ˈpækidɜːrmə]: literally "thick skin," also known as pachydermia. Unusually thick skin. When observed at the laryngeal level, pachyderma appears at the posterior glottis between the arytenoids and implies chronic reflux. (See **gastroesophageal reflux disease** and **laryngopharyngeal reflux,** 5.10 Reflux and Heartburn, and Figures 10.1a, 10.6a, 10.7b, 10.8, 10.12, and 15.3b.)

Papilloma [ˌpæpɪˈloʊmə]: also called papillomatosis and papillomata. Wart-like growths developing from exposure to any herpes-like virus. The growths are contagious, may recur unpredictably, and can spread. Of twenty-three varieties, #7 and #11 are laryngeal. Babies with infected mothers may catch the virus passing through the birth canal.

Paradoxical Vocal Fold Movement [ˌpærəˈdɑːksɪkl]: commonly called **vocal cord dysfunction**, although PVFM is a more current term. A disorder in which the vocal folds partially approximate on inhalation. May not only occur at the vocal fold level, but also at the epiglottic level in which the epiglottis constricts the airway. Abrupt onset is often triggered by reflux, due to a subconscious attempt to protect the trachea by narrowing the glottis and laryngeal vestibule, or can be triggered by stress. The disorder may worsen with exertion and displeasing smells. PVFM presents a wheeze on inhalation and shortness of breath and is commonly misdiagnosed as asthma. If you have been diagnosed with asthma and medications aren't working, it may be wise to consult a laryngologist to rule out PVFM. Checking for PVFM is a minor exam, whereas asthma can only be diagnosed by a doctor inducing it.

Paralysis [pəˈrælǝsɪs]: a complete inability to function due to nerve or muscular impairment. (See **vocal fold paralysis** and 10.16 Unilateral Vocal Fold Paralysis and Paresis.)

Paresis [pəˈrisǝs]: slight or partial paralysis, usually temporary and often caused by a virus. A vocal fold paresis is common and characterized by weakness, loss of muscle tone, and loss of mobility.

Passaggio [paˈsadʒɔ]: literally "passageway" or "bridge" in italian. The transitional pitch or consecutive pitches (usually two or three) that mark the end of one register and the beginning of another. Learning to manipulate this vocal transition has been compared to learning to shift gears in a standard car. The lengthener muscles/pitch muscles (cricothyroids) and the bulking muscles (thyroarytenoids) have a somewhat antagonistic relationship—kind of like biceps and triceps—in which one must relax for the other to contract. In the case of the thyroarytenoids and cricothyroids, however, both are employed in varying degrees, depending on where the singer is in her range and dynamic. When approaching the passaggio, the training singer will sense she is "hitting a ceiling" ascending in pitch or unable to descend further down the scale and an obvious break in phonation may occur. As singers gain coordination between developed vocal flexibility and breath support, these transitional areas between registers can become undetectable and seamless.

Pathogens [ˈpæθǝdʒǝnz]: substances capable of producing disease.

Pathology [pəˈθɑːlǝdʒi]: literally "reason for suffering." The name for any abnormality caused by disease. Physicians use the term to refer to anything that seems wrong or abnormal, as in "there is pathology in the larynx."

Pedunculated [pəˈdʌŋkjuleɪt]: literally "on a little foot." At the end of a stalk as in a pedunculated polyp.

Perimenopause [ˌperiˈmenǝpɔːz]: the time around menopause, including premenopause and the beginning of menopause. Perimenopause lasts an average of four years but can vary from six months to ten years.[5] Perimenopause begins as soon as cycle changes are observed (e.g., the days between periods shortens to every twenty-one to twenty-four days, rather than the usual twenty-eight to thirty days) and ends one year after the final menstrual period.

Period: when your vocal folds roll through one vibration (front to back, bottom to top), it's called a period.

Periodic: regular. In regard to the voice, periodic vibrations are vibrations that are consistent and symmetrical and occur with regularity. Periodic vibrations, as opposed to aperiodic vibrations, are a sign that the voice is healthy. They create a sound that we recognize as clean, pure, and even in tone and pitch.

Periodicity [ˌpɪriǝˈdɪsǝti]: how regular and consistent the vocal folds' vibratory pattern is.

Peripheral [pəˈrɪfǝrǝl]: situated in an outer, marginal boundary location, away from the center. May be used to refer to nerves outside the spinal cord or blood vessels outside the heart.

Petiole [ˈpetioʊl]: literally "little foot." The base of epiglottis.

Pharyngitis [ˌfærɪnˈdʒaɪtɪs]: literally "inflammation of the pharynx." Pharyngitis is the most common cause of a sore throat. Pharyngitis may be acute or chronic. Usually viral (won't respond to antibiotics and usually resolves on its own), but may also be bacterial (e.g., strep throat) or fungal infection (e.g., oral thrush/*Candida albicans*) or due to an environmental irritation.

---

5. Maude "Molly" Guerin, MD, Alliance Obstetrics and Gynecology, e-mail March 13, 2012.

Because symptoms for viral and bacterial pharyngitis are similar, diagnosis requires a throat swab (usually done only if white appears on tonsils, suggesting strep). Although a separate condition from laryngitis, pharyngitis may quickly lead to laryngitis as a secondary infection, in which case the vocal folds are likely to be affected. The common cold is a type of pharyngitis called nasopharyngitis and its drainage into the larynx often leads to a laryngeal infection. See **tonsillitis**.

Pharynx [ˈfærɪŋks]: plural: pharynges. A continuous muscular and membranous digestive tube and resonating space extending from behind the nose down the back of the mouth and into the larynx where it ends at the vocal folds and at the esophageal opening just posterior to the larynx.

Phonation: sound produced by vocal fold vibration.

Phonetic Symbols [fəˈnetɪk]: symbols representing sounds. The International Phonetic Alphabet (IPA) is not an alphabet of letters but of phonetic symbols. Speech-language pathologists (SLPs) and classically trained singers share a vast knowledge of phonetic symbols. SLPs learn IPA to communicate exact sounds heard in speech disorders, while classical singers use IPA to master the pronunciation of various foreign languages and to break down sounds for more understandable and healthier singing.

Phonosurgery: laryngeal surgery dealing with altering position, tension, mass, mobility, length, or shape of vocal folds to improve quality of voice. Phono- and microlaryngeal are the two types of vocal fold surgeries. All microlaryngeal vocal fold surgeries are phonosurgeries, but not all phonosurgeries are microlaryngeal. A laryngoplasty with Gore-Tex® and Silastic® medialization to correct vocal cord paralysis are phonosurgeries, for instance, that both require the surgeon to enter the larynx from the outside of the neck.

Phonotrauma: a preferable substitute for the term "vocal abuse" or "misuse" when talking with a patient.

Photocoagulation [ˌfoʊtoʊkoʊˌægjuˈleɪʃn]: a precise surgical technique using an intense, high-energy, fine-point beam of light from a laser to coagulate/clot or eliminate blood vessels by vaporizing them.

Physician: the only professional qualified and licensed to identify, medically diagnose, and prescribe treatment for pathology. A physician is not an expert on the behavioral aspects of pathology or the treatment realm, but mostly focuses on cutting and medicating. Examples are otolaryngologists. Pathologists are not physicians.

Phytochemical: a natural chemical compound found in plants.

Pink Noise: similar to and often mistakenly called **white noise**, but perhaps more pleasant to listen to, pink noise is composed of a wide range of frequencies sounding simultaneously and is found in nature. Examples are clapping or a crowd of people talking, the ocean, a waterfall, and a car or plane engine. Pink noise also masks other sounds well. Recordings of water are sold commercially to help relax people or even lull a baby to sleep.

Point of Maximum Glottal Contact: the area between 3 and 4 on the vocal folds, otherwise referred to as the junction of the anterior one third and the posterior two thirds of the vocal folds. This area takes the brunt of every vocal fold vibration, or more technically, the brunt of the folds' **lateral excursion**. See **lateral excursion**.

Polyp [ˈpɑːlɪp]: a bump resembling a blister in appearance that erupts from the basement membrane zone of the vocal fold epithelium. Broad-based/sessile types can be reabsorbed and go away. The skin tag/pedunculated types, however, will not and must be surgically removed.

Polypoid Corditis [ˈpɑːlɪpɔɪd kɔːrˈdaɪtəs]: also called polypoid degeneration and Reinke's edema. An abundance of thickened fluid in the superficial lamina propria that develops from regular overexposure to inhaled irritants (e.g., smokers) and those with severe reflux. The disorder will recur as long as one continues to be exposed to the irritant. Folds may thicken until they are so heavy that they get sucked in together on inhalation, making it difficult to breathe.

Posterior: toward the back, or behind.

Posterior Cricoarytenoid Muscles [ˌkraɪkoʊəˈrɪtənɔɪd]: the only muscles that abduct the folds.

Premenopause: the several years that precede menopause in which ovarian function wanes.

Presbylarynx [ˈprezbiˌlærɪŋks]: literally "old larynx." A condition of the larynx that can include any of the effects that aging has on the larynx and voice. (See 5.8 Old Age.)

Process [ˈprɑːses]: a section of bone or tissue that projects out. The body has many including the muscular and vocal processes of the arytenoid cartilages.

Prosection: a cadaver or anatomical part that has been precut by an experienced anatomist to isolate a specific structure for easy access and quick study. Prosection is valuable for teaching anatomy and techniques used in surgery.

Protein-Bound Water: fluid that is replenished by long-term hydration and mobilized only by hormonal shifts and steroids, not diuretics or other means.

Puberphonia [ˌpjuːbərˈfoʊniə]: also known as mutational falsetto, incomplete mutation, and adolescent transitional dysphonia. A persistent high, breathy falsetto in a male (and occasionally a female) past puberty and with a seemingly normal larynx. Commonly stems from a psychological disorder or learned behavior. Physiological causes such as an endocrine imbalance are rare and must be ruled out.

Pyriform Sinus [ˈpirɪfɔrm]: two deep laryngeal spaces located between the larynx and esophagus that help protect the airway by acting as gutters for collecting mucus. Their contents spill into the esophagus as the larynx rises with swallowing. They can overcontract with mtd. Cancer that develops in these sinuses is called silent cancer and almost always requires a complete laryngectomy due to its late diagnosis. Until the lesion has matured (i.e., embedding itself in muscle and large enough to interfere with swallowing), it goes undetected.

R

Reactive change: any change produced as a result of an outside influence. Voice specialists often use this term when referring to the effects that a unilateral lesion may have on the opposite fold.

Rebound Hypoglycemia [ˌhaɪpoʊɡlaɪˈsiːmiə]: a condition where a lack of blood sugar causes acute fatigue, irritability, and weakness.

Recurrent Laryngeal Nerve [ləˈrɪndʒiəl]: controls all the intrinsic laryngeal muscles except the cricothyroid.

Re-epithelialization [riˌepɪˌθiliəlˈzeɪʃn]: epithelial tissue regrowth over a wound in epithelium.

Reflux: when food, liquid, or acid contents from the stomach leak back into the esophagus.

Reflux Laryngitis [ˌlærɪnˈdʒaɪtɪs]: laryngitis caused by regurgitation of stomach acid into the pharynx and onto the arytenoid mucosa and posterior vocal folds. The gastric acid burns laryngeal tissue, causing it to redden and swell.

Reinke's Space [ˈreɪŋkiz]: the superficial layer of the lamina propria was discovered by a man by the name of Reinke and has historically been referred to as Reinke's space. Because the layer isn't an empty space at all, the term "superficial lamina propria" is preferred.

Residual Air: air that still remains in the lungs even after complete exhalation. Ten percent of our TLV is reserved for residual air that doesn't leave our lungs until we die.

Resonating Cavity: also called resonator. A space through which a sound wave directly travels. The cavities through which a human voice can resonate are the pharynx (including the nasopharynx, oropharynx, and laryngopharynx), the mouth, the nose, and, to a small degree, the sinuses.

Rhinology [raɪˈnɑːlədʒi]: a subspecialization of otolaryngology, like laryngology, but the study of the nose and sinuses.

Rigid Fiberoptic Oral Endoscope [ˌfaɪbərˈɑːptɪk ˈendəskoʊp]: the instrument used to view the larynx via the mouth. The long metal rod contains a bundle of light strands that illuminate the larynx for viewing and recording purposes.

Rigid Laryngoscope [læˈrɪŋgəskoʊp]: see **rigid fiberoptic oral endoscope.**

S

Sagittal [ˈsædʒɪtl]: an anatomical view via a vertical/longitudinal cut.

Sanitization: "the process of chemical or mechanical cleansing, applicable in public health systems.... It reduces microbes ... to safe, acceptable levels for public health."[6]

Serous [ˈsɪrəs]: having a thin, watery consistency.

Serum [ˈsɪrəm]: Latin for "whey." A thin, clear, and yellowish fluid primarily made up of water and produced in the body's bloodstream and that separates when the blood clots. The word derives from the liquid that separates from the curd when making cheese. Serum can also be used to refer to any serum-type fluid, such as that found in a blister. Serum is just a carrier for the substances needed to fight infection and help heal injuries. Serum collects at wounded or irritated sites, making them edematous.

Sessile [ˈsesl]: as opposed to pedunculated, attached directly by a broad base.

Shimmer: an increase or decrease in amplitude.

Singer's Formant: a 2,500-HZ to 3,500-HZ "ring" in the voice thought to be produced by contracting and thus narrowing the aryepiglottic sphincter. (See 14.3 How are Opera Singers Heard Over an Orchestra Without Amplification?)

Sjögren's Syndrome [ˈSoʊgrɪnz]: an autoimmune disorder that destroys the mucus- and tear-producing glands in the body. This disorder can develop on its own (primary) or out of a preexisting condition, such as rheumatoid arthritis (secondary), and may require medications that suppress the immune system. One may experience a few symptoms of the disorder without having the disease. In such cases, the symptoms are usually very treatable.

Skeletal Muscle: muscles that attach to bones or cartilages to support the skeleton. Skeletal muscle contraction is controlled consciously. The majority of the muscles in the body are skeletal muscle. They have a point of origin and a point of insertion and shorten with

---

6 Sridhar Rao, PN, "Sterilization and Disinfection," June 2008, http://www.microrao.com/micronotes/steriliza-tion.pdf, accessed January 15, 2010.

contraction, pulling toward their point of origin. They also work in pairs, so that one must relax for the other to contract (e.g., biceps and triceps). See **muscular antagonism**.

Sleep Apnea [æpˈniːə]: also called obstructive sleep apnea syndrome (OSAS). A disease suffered by children and adults characterized by hypernasality, loud snoring, restless sleep, and labored respiration during sleep caused by airway obstruction.

Smooth Muscle: muscles found in the walls of hollow organs. Smooth muscle contracts without conscious control, and its contraction makes the organ smaller. They are uniquely elastic and able to contract while being stretched, which is crucial for uterine, urinary bladder, and intestinal function. They are found in many other places in the body as well, such as the iris of the eye, arteries, and veins.

Soft Palate: also called the **muscular palate**. The soft tissue portion of the roof of the mouth that begins where the bony hard palate ends at the back of the oral cavity. The soft palate is a layered fold of tissue, including a layer of muscle that plays a role in swallowing, articulating, and forming vowels and resonance. It relaxes during passive respiration and elevates for swallowing (to prevent food from entering the nose) and yawning. See **velum**.

Spasmodic Dysphonia [spæzˈmɑːdɪk dɪsˈfoʊniə]: a disorder characterized by tight, strangled-sounding phonation due to extreme laryngeal tension. There are two possible types of laryngeal tension involved: the tightening of muscles in adduction (spasms of hypercompression) or abduction (spasms of hypocompression). Spasms of hypocompression are more common in women, especially those over forty-five years. Talking on the phone is the hardest means of communication. Yelling is easiest. Condition worsens with emotional stress. Diagnosis is reached through a team of doctors eliminating what it isn't. This team includes an SLP, a neurologist, and a laryngologist. There is no cure, but symptoms may improve with periodic BOTOX® injections, vocal rehabilitation, or, in the case of hypercompression, the surgical crushing of the recurrent nerve (not an option in hypocompression patients because they wouldn't be able to breathe). See **botulism**.

Speech-Language Pathologist [pəˈθɑːlədʒɪst]: synonymous with voice pathologist, speech therapist, and speech pathologist. SLPs are experts in speech and voice disorders with specialized training in strobovideolaryngoscopy and thus qualified to perform, but not interpret, strobovideolaryngoscopy exams. More so than physicians, SLPs are experts in the behavioral and treatment aspects of voice pathology. (See 6.2 The Voice Specialists.)

Sphincter [ˈsfɪŋktər]: a circular band of muscle that contracts to close an entrance. The body has many sphincters including the upper and lower esophageal sphincters, the rectal sphincter, and the aryepiglottic sphincter of the larynx. The latter doesn't actually close, but tightens to protectively narrow the space above the vocal folds during swallowing.

Squamous Debris [ˈskweməs deˈbri]: loose particles of scaly tissue.

Stenosis [steˈnoʊsəs]: narrowing. Results mostly from scar tissue formation.

Stoma: the window cut that is made into the trachea during a tracheostomy.

Strap muscles: four muscles that look like straps in the front of the neck that connect to the outside of the larynx. Their contraction lowers the larynx for swallowing and some speaking and singing.

Stratified Squamous Epithelium [ˈstrætɪfaɪd ˈskweməsˌepɪˈθiliəm]: comes from Greek *strategos*, meaning "general" (as in a rank in the army), and specifies a tissue made up of tightly bound scale-like cell layers. Designed to cover surfaces needing physical protection and can be with or without keratin, a tough protein. Keratinized stratified squamous epithelium includes the skin and tongue. Nonkeratinized-type surfaces include the esophagus, vagina, and true vocal folds (which endure high impact during vibration).

Stridor [ˈstraɪdər]: inhalation noises caused by airway obstruction.

Stroboscopy [strouˈbɑːskəpi]: a laryngeal examination in which a strobe light is used during a laryngoscopy exam to observe vocal fold function. (See **video laryngeal stroboscopy** and 8.3 Instruments Used in the Clinic.)

Subclavian Artery [sʌbˈkleɪviən]: two major arteries of the chest that mainly supply the right and left arms with blood.

Subspecialize: to specialize further by pursuing education in an even narrower field of study within a specialty.

Subglottal: adj. Meaning below the glottis. The area of the larynx below the true vocal folds including the cricoid cartilage and trachea.

Sublingual [sʌbˈlɪŋgwəl]: adj. Meaning below the tongue.

Sulcus Vergeture [ˈvərgɪtʃər]: sulcus literally means "a groove" and vergeture "a linear stretch mark." An acquired dip in the vocal fold developed from the cover binding to the ligament underneath.

Superior: above or upper.

Superior Laryngeal Nerve [ləˈrɪndʒiəl]: the superior laryngeal nerve of the vagus has two branches—the external, which controls the cricothyroid muscle (e.g., tells cricothyroid muscle to elongate to create a higher pitch), and the internal, which enters the larynx and supplies sensation to the laryngeal mucosa (e.g., causes the tickle that provokes a cough when it detects foreign substances).

Supraglottal: adj. Meaning above the **glottis**. The area of the larynx above the true folds.

Supraglottis: anatomical term for the area of the larynx above the true vocal folds and below the hyoid bone, including the ventricular and aryepiglottic folds, the epiglottis, the arytenoid cartilages, and the walls of the hypopharynx.

T

Temporomandibular Joint [ˌtempəroʊmænˈdɪbjulər]: abbr. TMJ, literally "temple" (bone at the side of the head), "mandible" (lower jaw), "joint" (the point of two of more bones coming together that permits or prevents motion of either or both bones). The TMJ is a *ginglymo* (hinge) *arthrodial* (limited movement in all directions) joint and functions much like the hinge on a door. It is a *synovial* joint, meaning that the joint cavity is made slippery with a raw egg white–like fluid.

Temporomandibular Joint Dysfunction [ˌtempəroʊmænˈdɪbjulər]: abbr. TMD, also called temporomandibular joint disorder. A joint disorder often characterized by painful clicking, popping, and limited movement of the jaw. Generally stems from constant excessive pressure due to teeth grinding, faulty bite, habitual teeth clenching, and pushing the tongue against the roof of mouth and is aggravated by chewing. If the joint is damaged, the disc that cushions the joint may slip out of place and cause the jaw to lock open or shut. Surgery to fix the disc comes with its own problems and is not recommended. Physical therapy may help to recapture the disc and maintain proper disc positioning. Steroid injections can help to decrease stiffness and pain. A custom-made bite guard that is specially designed to fit over the lower teeth and correct your alignment can be worn at night to support the joint and alleviate discomfort.

Tendon: tough, nonelastic bands that attach muscles to bone.

Tessitura [tesi'tura]: four or five neighboring pitches where the voice is most comfortable singing. We apply this singing term to the speaking voice as well. The tessitura for the speaking and singing voices will likely be different.

Thermal Damage: injury caused by heat (i.e., burns).

Thoracic cavity [θɔːˈræsɪk]: the upper chamber of the torso that contains the heart and lungs. Also called chest cavity.

Thoracic Fixation [θɔːˈræsɪk]: also called **Valsalva maneuver.** A major function of the laryngeal mechanism in which the true and false vocal folds close and trap and forcibly hold air in the lungs. You can experience thoracic fixation by attempting to exhale while you hold your breath. The increased pressure placed on the abdomen helps us to vomit, defecate, give birth, cough, and lift heavy objects.

Thyroarytenoid Muscles [ˌθaɪroʊəˈrɪtənɔɪd]: two bundles of muscles (the vocalis and the thyromuscularis) that extend from behind and below the thyroid notch to slightly different points on the arytenoid cartilages. The vocalis forms the body of the true vocal folds. The vocalis contracts (shortening) for lower pitches and tensing the folds to achieve full glottal closure.

Thyroid Cartilage [ˈθaɪrɔɪd]: literally "shield-like." The thyroid cartilage is the largest of the laryngeal cartilages. This cartilage is shaped like a shield and helps to protect the vocal folds and upper airway. The vocal folds connect to the thyroid cartilage anteriorly.

Thyroid notch [ˈθaɪrɔɪd]: the dip at the top of the thyroid cartilage prominence.

Thyroplasty [ˈθaɪroʊˌplæsti]: a surgical alteration of the larynx to improve voicing. Also called laryngeal framework surgery.

Tidal Volume: the sum total of air inhaled and exhaled during one passive respiratory cycle.

Tissue: structurally and functionally similar cells that function as a unit.

Titrate: to determine an appropriate dosage by taking a lower dosage of a medication than what is recommended and gradually adding more and adjusting until the desired effect is reached.

Tonsillar Pillars: also called palatine [ˈpælətaɪn] arches, faucial [ˈfɔːʃl] pillars. Bilateral vertical mucosal tissue extending down from the soft palate at the sides of the oropharynx and coming down on either side of the palatine tonsils (a.k.a. faucial tonsils).

Tonsillitis: literally "inflammation of the tonsils." Tonsillitis is a type of chronic or acute, viral or bacterial pharyngitis and is also called pharyngotonsillitis or tonsillopharyngitis. An inflamed soft palate will be painful to raise/vault when singing. May lead to and occur in tandem with laryngitis. Inflamed tonsils may enlarge enough to alter the feel of singing and even obstruct the airway. If the tonsillitis threatens the airway, or if it is chronic and doesn't respond to other treatments, the tonsils will need to be surgically removed. (See **tonsils** and **tonsillar pillars**, and Tonsillitis in 12.3 Common Problems Where Surgery Could Affect the Vocal Mechanism.)

Tonsils: Latin for "almond." Rounded lymphatic tissue. There are three sets of tonsils: the lingual tonsils at the very back of the tongue, between the base of the tongue and the epiglottis; the palatine tonsils (a.k.a. faucial tonsils) at the sides of the oropharynx that are partially surrounded by the **tonsillar pillars**; and the adenoids (a.k.a. pharyngeal tonsils) at the junction of the pharynx and the nose. Tonsil function is uncertain but they are believed to produce antibodies that help prevent respiratory infections.

Topical Anesthetic: see **anesthesia.**

Total Lung Capacity: the total amount of air that lungs hold. The average adult lungs hold about six liters of air in females and seven liters of air in males.[7] Not all of this air is available for use and some doesn't leave the lungs until we die. See **residual volume**.

Total Lung Volume: consists of a person's vital capacity (roughly four to five liters in the average adult) and residual volume (approximately two liters), which is never depleted unless lungs collapse.

Trachea ['treɪkiə]: a cartilaginous and membranous tube that averages 4 inches in length and is only as big around as an index finger. All the air that passes in and out of the body travels through this small tube. It extends from the bottom of the larynx and branches into two tubes called bronchi just before entering the lungs. Known commonly as the windpipe.

Tracheostomy [ˌtreɪkiˈɑːstəmi]: also called tracheotomy. A surgical procedure in which an opening (**stoma**) is made into the trachea below the cricoid cartilage at the base of the neck.

Transverse: anatomical plane of reference implying a cut that divides an object into top and bottom.

Transverse Arytenoid Muscle: see **interarytenoideus**.

Trauma: injury.

Turbinates ['tɜːrbɪnəts]: also called turbinate bones or nasal conchae. The turbinates are three paired and scroll-shaped bony projections inside each nasal cavity that are covered by mucous membrane. Air travels through the spaces (meatus) above and below them when you breathe.

U

Ulcerations [ʌlsəˈreɪʃnz]: inflammatory breakdown of the skin that leaves raw sores.

Unilateral [ˌjuːnɪˈlætrəl]: only on one side.

Upper esophageal sphincter [iˈsɑːfədʒiːl ˈsfɪŋktər]: the upper portion of the esophagus. The ues contains a ring-like muscle that acts similarly to a one-way valve, allowing food and water to pass into the esophagus upon swallowing and inhibiting food from coming back up into the pharynx. See **esophageal sphincter**.

Uvula ['juːvjələ]: literally "little grape" in Latin; also called palatine uvula. The small dangling membrane of mucosa-covered tissue that hangs down from the soft palate. Like the tonsils, the uvula is a lymph node, or an interr'ogation spot for bacteria, screening the bacteria and providing antibodies to help fend off respiratory infection.

Uvulectomy [juːvjəˈlektəmi]: surgical excision of the uvula.

Uvulopalatopharyngoplasty [ˌjuːvjuːloʊˌpælətoʊ fæˈrɪŋgoʊˌplæsti]: a surgical procedure used to remove tissue in the throat. Also called UPPP or UP3, this surgery is commonly used for patients with obstructive sleep apnea who cannot tolerate continuous positive airway pressure (CPAP) therapy. It can involve the removal of the uvula, soft palate, tonsils, adenoids, and pharynx.

V

Vagus ['veɪgəs]: also called cranial nerve #10 or CN X because it is the tenth of twelve cranial nerves. It is a major nerve and also called a parent nerve because it gives off many smaller nerves

---

[7] J. Stocks and Ph. H. Quanjer, "Reference Values for Residual Volume, Functional Residual Capacity, and Total Lung Capacity," *European Respiration Journal* 8 (1995): 492–506.

(like the SLN and RLN) in order to innervate the external ear, some taste buds, the pharynx, the larynx, the esophagus, the heart, the intestines, and most other abdominal organs.

Vallecula [və-'le-kyə-lə]: shallow dip or indentation such as the furrow separating the two hemispheres of the brain. With regard to the larynx, the vallecula describes the "little valley" between the epiglottis and tongue.

Valsalva Maneuver: see **thoracic fixation.**

Varix ['verɪks]: (plural: varices) any prominent blood vessel. In the varicose vein family. Often appears as a tiny "pepper speck" or "pinpoint" capillary prominence on the vocal fold.

Vascular ['væskjələr]: pertaining to blood vessels. When used to describe an organ or tissue, the term "vascular" may indicate a heavy supply of blood vessels.

Velum ['viːləm]: literally "veil." Refers specifically to the free edge of the soft palate from which the uvula hangs at its center. Also refers to any thin partition or covering in the body. (See Figure 8.5c.)

Ventricle ['ventrɪkl]: any small recess or hollow space. In regards to the larynx, the ventricle is the space above each true vocal fold and below each false vocal fold. Both spaces must be unobstructed for the true vocal folds to vibrate freely.

Venule ['vinyuːl]: Latin for "little vein," also called venula. Venules are the smallest veins and are connected to the smallest arteries (arterioles) by the tiniest blood vessels (capillaries). The larynx contains venules and capillaries only. No arterioles, arteries, or veins.

Vestibule ['vestɪbjuːl]: a cavity or chamber that leads to or is another entrance to an additional cavity or space.

Vestibular Ligament [ves'tɪbjuːlər]: the strong band of fibrous tissue within the false vocal folds.

Vibrate: to make a fast succession of regular or irregular oscillations or movements.

Video Laryngeal Stroboscopy [lə'rɪndʒiəl stroʊ'baːskəpi]: video imaging of the vocal folds moving in simulated slow motion. See **stroboscopy.**

Viscera ['vɪsərə]: plural of viscus (meaning an internal organ). The organs contained in the body's cavities, especially those in the abdomen (the lower esophagus, stomach, intestines, liver, spleen, pancreas, colon, kidneys, gallbladder, bladder, duodenum, jejunum, ileum, cecum, appendix, and rectum).

Viscous ['vɪskəs]: having sticky, glue-like properties.

Vocal Abuse: generally speaking, any vocal behavior that is harmful to the vocal folds. This book differentiates between harmful behaviors that are one-time occurrences (**vocal misuses**) and those that are habitual (vocal abuses) such as phonation that is pitched too low or too loud, voice overuse, and hard glottal onsets. Among clinicians, the two terms are loosely interchangeable. Some advocate getting rid of both classifications in favor of the gentler and more generic term "phonotrauma," especially when speaking with patients.

Vocal Folds: two separate folds of layered tissues that come together over the trachea and vibrate to produce sound. The false vocal folds are located above the true vocal folds and do not take part in phonation.

Vocal Cord Dysfunction [ˌpærə'daːksɪkl]: see **paradoxical vocal fold movement.**

Vocal Fold Paralysis: complete interruption of nerve impulses to the muscles that control laryngeal movement. A paralysis can affect one or both vocal folds. Vocal folds can paralyze in any position from totally adducted to totally abducted. Depending on the position of fixation, the patient may experience problems with voice, breathing, and/or swallowing. (See **paralysis** and 10.16 Unilateral Vocal Fold Paralysis and Paresis.)

Vocal Hyperfunction: opposite of vocal hypofunction. Increased adduction of the vocal folds resulting in reduced airflow during phonation. The resulting sound may be strained or "pressed."

Vocal Hypofunction: reduced approximation of the vocal folds resulting in excessive breathiness. Hypofunctional voice problems can range from mild breathiness to complete aphonia (whisper) and may be structural (i.e., paralysis or age-related bowing) or functional (i.e., psychological, behavioral).

Vocal Ligament: a strong band of elastic tissue within the true vocal folds and the false vocal folds.

Vocal Misuse: generally speaking, any vocal behavior that is harmful to the vocal folds. This book differentiates between harmful behaviors that are one-time occurrences (vocal misuses) such as one big yell or scream and those that are habitual (vocal abuses). Among clinicians, the two terms are loosely interchangeable. Some advocate getting rid of both classifications in favor of the gentler and more generic term "phonotrauma," especially when speaking with patients.

Vocal Onset: the initiation of vocal fold phonation. The moment voicing or vibration of the vocal folds begins.

Vocal Process: the anterior projection of the arytenoid cartilage to which the vocal ligament attaches. There are two, one on each arytenoid.

Vocal Tract: the vocal tract is made up of all your resonating cavities, in other words, all the spaces directly accessible to the sound waves traveling up from your vocal folds. As the sound waves leave the vocal folds, they enter spaces available to them and resonate in those spaces. The vocal tract consists of the laryngeal vestibule, the pharynx (the laryngopharynx, oropharynx, and nasopharynx), the oral cavity, the nasal cavity, and the sinus cavities.

Voice Clinic: commonly associated with a facility where a team of professionals evaluate and treat voice disorders. Many voice clinics also conduct voice research and provide educational outreach pertaining to voice.

Voice Pedagogue ['pedəgɑːg]: a person who specializes in and teaches the art, science, method, and practice of singing.

Voice Therapy: the treatment of vocal dysfunction or injury by use of therapeutic exercises intended to restore or facilitate normal function or development. Voice therapy may also be needed to decrease the size of a lesion and reduce inflammation before surgery.

W

White Noise: a noise that consists of all frequencies sounding simultaneously at the same energy level, including those not perceived by the human ear. True white noise can only be produced by a special generator. White noise easily masks other sounds and, depending on the volume, can make it difficult for you to hear your own voice. White noise generators are available commercially and sometimes used by employers to help create a better working environment. Naturally occurring sounds that come close to white noise are a hiss and radio or tv static. (These examples, however, are still pink noise.)

X

Xenon Light [ˈziːnɑːn]: also called xenon lamp. An artificially produced light using ionized xenon gas to mimic natural daylight. Most true strobe lighting uses xenon. Xenon is expensive but is the best option for high-intensity lighting needed for short durations. The lamp can burn for 2,000 hours.

BIBLIOGRAPHY

CONFERENCE PAPERS AND SEMINARS

Cristoloveanu, Carmen, M. Ramez Salem, and Ninos J. Joseph. "Does Positioning the Upper End of the Tracheal Tube Cuff 2 cm Below the Vocal Cords Assure Proper Tracheal Tube Insertion Depth?" Paper presented at the annual meeting for the American Society of Anesthesiologists, San Diego, California, October 16–20, 2010.

BOOKS

Baken, Ronald J., and Robert F. Orlikoff. *Clinical Measurement of Speech and Voice*. San Diego: Singular, 2000.

Baum, Gerald L., James D. Crapo, Bartolome R. Celli, and Joel B. Karlinsky, eds. *Textbook of Pulmonary Diseases*, Volume 1. Philadelphia: Lippincott-Raven, 1998.

Benninger, M. S. *Vocal Arts Medicine: The Care and Prevention of Professional Voice Disorders*. New York: Thieme Medical Publishers, 1994.

Boldrey, Richard. *Guide to Operatic Roles & Arias*. Dallas: Pst ... Inc., 1994.

Clark, Nancy. *Sports Nutrition Guidebook*, 2nd ed. Brookline, MA: Sports Medicine Systems, 1997.

Columbus Dietetic Association, ed. *Manual of Clinical Dietetics*. Columbus, OH: Old Trail Printing, 1991.

Dawkins, Richard. *The Greatest Show on Earth: The Evidence for Evolution*. New York: Free Press, 2009.

McCoy, Scott. *Your Voice: An Inside View*. Princeton, NJ: Inside View Press, 2004.

Miller, Richard. *Training Soprano Voices*. New York: Oxford University Press, 2000.

University of California at Berkeley, ed. *The New Wellness Encyclopedia*. Boston: Houghton Mifflin, 1995.

CHAPTERS IN BOOKS

Benninger, Michael S. "Medical Disorders in the Vocal Artist." In *Vocal Arts Medicine: The Care and Prevention of Professional Voice Disorders*, edited by Michael S. Benninger. New York: Thieme Medical Publishers, 1994.

Columbus Dietetic Association, ed. "Nutrition for the Athlete." In *Manual of Clinical Dietetics*. Columbus, OH: Old Trail Printing, 1991.

Ford, Charles N. "Phonosurgery." In *Vocal Arts Medicine: The Care and Prevention of Professional Voice Disorders*, edited by Michael S. Benninger, 344–355. New York: Thieme Medical Publishers, 1994.

Sataloff, Robert T., Joseph Sataloff, and Caren J. Sokolow. "Hearing Loss in Musicians." In *Occupational Hearing Loss*, 3rd ed., edited by Robert Thayer Sataloff and Joseph Sataloff, 718–729. Boca Raton: CRC Press, 2006.

Thurman, Leon, and Carol Klitzke. "How Vocal Abilities Can Be Enhanced by Nutrition and Body Movement." In *Bodymind and Voice: Foundations of Voice Education*, edited by Leon Thurman and Graham Welch, 433–441. Iowa City: National Center for Voice and Speech, 1997.

Thurman, Leon, Carol Klitzke, and Norman Hogikyan. "Cornerstones of Voice Protection." In *Bodymind and Voice: Foundations of Voice Education*, edited by Leon Thurman and Graham Welch, 442–451. Iowa City: National Center for Voice and Speech, 1997.

Thurman, Leon, Axel Theimer, Graham Welch, Elizabeth Grefsheim, and Patricia Feit. "Creating Breathflow for Skilled Speaking and Singing." In *Bodymind and Voice: Foundations of Voice Education*, edited by Leon Thurman and Graham Welch, 156–172. Iowa City: National Center for Voice and Speech, 1997.

Thurman, Leon, Graham Welch, Axel Theimer, Patricia Feit, and Elizabeth Grefsheim. "What Your Larynx Does When Vocal Sounds Are Created." In *Bodymind and Voice: Foundation of Voice Education*, edited by Leon Thurman and Graham Welch, 186. Iowa City: National Center for Voice and Speech, 1997.

ARTICLES

Abitbol, Jean, Patrick Abitbol, and Beatrice Abitbol. "Sex Hormones and the Female Voice." *Journal of Voice* 13, no. 3 (September 1999): 424–446.

Abitbol, Jean, Jean de Brux, Ginette Millot, Marie-Francoise Masson, Odile Languille Mimoun, Helene Pau, and Beatrice Abitbol. "Does a Hormonal Vocal Cord Cycle Exist in Women? Study of Vocal Premenstrual Syndrome in Voice Performers by Videostroboscopy-Glottography and Cytology on 38 Women." *Journal of Voice* 3, no. 2 (1989): 157–162.

Ayres, J. G., E. D. Bateman, B. Lundback, and T. A. J. Harris. "High Dose Fluticasone Propionate,1 mg Daily, Versus Fluticasone Propionate, 2 mg Daily, or Budesonide, 1.6 mg Daily, in Patients With Chronic Severe Asthma." *European Respiratory Journal* 8 (1995): 579–586.

Banks, Siobhan, and David F. Dinges. "Behavioral and Physiological Consequences of Sleep Restriction." *Journal of Clinical Sleep Medicine* 3, no. 5 (August 15, 2007): 519–528.

Blomgren, Michael, Yang Chen, Manwa L. Ng, and Harvey R. Gilbert. "Acoustic, Aerodynamic, Physiologic, and Perceptual Properties of Modal and Vocal Fry Registers." *Journal of Acoustical Society of America* 103, no. 5 (May 1998): 2649–2658.

Bodger, K., and N. Trudgill. "Guidelines for Oesophageal Manometry and pH Monitoring." *BSC Guidelines in Gastroenterology*, November 2006, 1–10.

Breatnach, Eamann, Gypsy C. Abbott, and Robert G. Fraser. "Dimensions of the Normal Human Trachea." *American Journal of Roentgenology* 141 (May 1983): 903–906.

Brodsky, Jay B., Alex Macario, and James B. D. Mark. "Tracheal Diameter Predicts Double-Lumen Tube Size: A Method for Selecting Left Double-Lumen Tubes." *Anesthesia & Analgesia* 82, no. 4 (April 1996): 861–864.

Casa, Douglas J., Lawrence E. Armstrong, Susan K. Hillman, Scott J. Montain, Ralph V. Reiff, Brent S. E. Rich, William O. Roberts, and Jennifer A. Stone. "National Athletic Trainers' Association Position Statement: Fluid Replacement for Athletes." *Journal of Athletic Training* 35, no. 2 (June 2000): 212–224.

Chae, Sung Won, G. Choi, H. J. Kang, J. O. Choi, and S. M. Jin. "Clinical Analysis of Voice Change as a Parameter of Premenstrual Syndrome." *Journal of Voice* 15, no. 2 (June 2001): 278–283.

Chae, Sung Won, Geon Choi, Hee Joon Kang, Jong Ouck Choi, and Sung Min Jin. "Clinical Analysis of Voice Change as a Parameter of Premenstrual Syndrome." *Journal of Voice* 15, no. 2 (June 2001): 278–283.

Clark, D. J., and B. J. Lipworth. "Adrenal Suppression With Chronic Dosing of Fluticasone Propionate Compared With Budesonide in Adult Asthmatic Patients." *Thorax* 52 (1997): 55–58.

Fabbri, L., P. S. Burge, L. Croonenborgh, F. Warlies, B. Weeke, A. Ciaccia, and C. Parker. "Comparison of Fluticasone Propionate With Beclomethasone Disproportionate in Moderate to Severe Asthma Treated for One Year." *Thorax* 48 (1993): 817–823.

Folprechtova, A., and O. Miksovska. "The Acoustic Conditions in a Symphony Orchestra." *Pracov Lek* 28 (1978): 1–2.

Gelfer, M. P., M. L. Andrews, and C. P. Schmidt. "Documenting Laryngeal Change Following Prolonged Loud Reading." *Journal of Voice* 10 (1996): 368–377.

Giovanni, A., C. Chanteret, and A. Lagler. "Sulcus Vocalis: A Review." *European Archives Otorhinolaryngology Journal* 264, no. 4 (April 2007): 337–344.

Grandjean, Ann C., Kristin J. Reimers, Karen E. Bannick, and Mary C. Haven. "The Effect of Caffeinated, Non-Caffeinated, Caloric and Non-Caloric Beverages on Hydration." *Journal of the American College of Nutrition* 19, no. 5 (2000): 591–600.

Harding, S. M. "The Human Pharmacology of Fluticasone Propionate." *Respiratory Medicine* 84, Suppl. A (1990): 25–29.

Hirano, Miranu. "Vocal Mechanisms in Singing: Laryngological and Phoniatric Aspects" Journal of Voice 2, no.1 (1988): 51–69.

Jahn, Anthony. "Vitamins and Herbal Medicines: All Good?" *Classical Singer*, December 2001, 22.

Johnson, L. F., and T. R. DeMeester. "Twenty-Four Hour pH Monitoring of the Distal Esophagus: A Quantitative Measure of Gastroesophageal Reflux." *American Journal of Gastroenterology* 62, no. 4 (1974): 325–332.

Lã, Filipa, and Jane W. Davidson. "Investigating the Relationship Between Sexual Hormones and Female Western Classical Singing." *Research Studies in Music Education* 24 (June 2005): 75–87. doi:10.1177/1321103X050240010601.

Lacina, V. "Der Einfluss der Menstruation auf die Stimme der Sängerinnen." *Folia Phoniatrica* 20 (1968): 13–24.

Leydon, Ciara, Marcin Wroblewski, Naomi Eichorn, and Mahalakshmi Sivasankar. "A Meta-Analysis of Outcomes of Hydration Intervention on Phonation Threshold Pressure." *Journal of Voice* 24, no. 6 (November 2010): 637–643.

Lombard, Étienne. "Le signe de l'élévation de la voix." *Annales des Maladies de L'Oreille et du Larynx* 37, no. 2 (1911): 101–119.

Mantgomery, W. W. "Cricoarytenoid Arthritis." *The Laryngoscope* 73, no. 7 (2009): 801–836.

Maughan, R. J., and J. Griffin. "Caffeine Ingestion and Fluid Balance: A Review." *Journal of Human Nutrition and Dietetics* 16, no. 6 (2003): 411–420. doi:10.1046/j.1365–277X.2003.00477.x.

Miller, K. W. P., P. L. Walker, and R. L. O'Halloran. "Age and Sex-Related Variation in Hyoid Bone Morphology." *Journal of Forensic Science* 43, no. 6 (1998): 1138–1143.

Miller, Vanessa L., Michael Stewart, and Mark Lehman. "Noise and Hearing Loss in Musicians." *Medical Problems of Performing Artists,* December 2007, 160–165.

Papadopoulos, N., G. Lykaki-Anastopoulou, and El. Alvanidou. "The Shape and Size of the Human Hyoid Bone and a Proposal for an Alternative Classification." *Journal of Anatomy* 163 (1989): 249–260.

Santos, P. M., A. Afrassiabi, and E. A. Weymuller Jr. "Risk Factors Associated With Prolonged Intubation and Laryngeal Injury." *Otolaryngology—Head and Neck Surgery* 111, no. 4 (October 1994): 453–459.

Sato, K., S. Kurita, M. Hirano, and K. Kiyokawa. "Distribution of Elastic Cartilage in the Arytenoids and Its Physiologic Significance." *Annals of Otology, Rhinology, and Laryngology* 99, 5 Pt. 1 (May 1990): 363–368.

Solomon, N. P., and M. S. DiMattia. "Effects of a Vocally Fatiguing Task and Systemic Hydration on Phonation Threshold Pressure." *Journal of Voice* 14 (2000): 341–362.

Solomon, N. P., Leslie E. Glaze, Robert R. Arnold, and Miriam van Mersbergen. "Effects of a Vocally Fatiguing Task and Systemic Hydration on Men's Voices." *Journal of Voice* 17 (March 2003): 31–46.

Spirling, Lucy I., and Ian R. Daniels. "Peppermint: More Than Just an After-Dinner Mint." *Journal of the Royal Society for the Promotion of Health* 121 (March 2001): 62–63. Accessed August 14, 2011. doi:10.1177/146642400112100113.

Stemple, J., J. Stanley, and L. Lee. "Objective Measures of Voice Production in Normal Subjects Following Prolonged Voice Use." *Journal of Voice* 9 (1995): 127–133.

Stocks, J., and P. H. Quanjer. "Reference Values for Residual Volume, Functional Residual Capacity, and Total Lung Capacity." *European Respiratory Journal* 8 (1995): 492–506. Accessed June 25, 2012. doi:10.1183/09031936.95.08030492.

Tutuian, Radu, and Donald O. Castell. "Gastroesophageal Reflux Monitoring: pH and Impedance." *GI Motility online,* May 2006. Accessed August 22, 2011. doi:10.1038/gimo31.

Xue, Steve A., and Jianping G. Hao. "Normative Standards for Vocal Tract Dimensions by Race as Measured by Acoustic Pharyngometry." *Journal of Voice* 20, no. 3 (September 2006): 391–400.

WEBSITES

American Speech-Language-Hearing Association (ASHA). "Vocal Tract Visualization and Imaging: Position Statement." PS2004–00121. Accessed August 8, 2012. http://www.asha.org/policy. doi:10.1044/policy.

Centers for Disease Control and Prevention. "Annual Smoking-Attributable Mortality, Years of Potential Life Lost, and Economic Costs—United States, 1995–1999." *Morbidity and Mortality Weekly Report* 51, 14 (2002): 300–303. Accessed July 24, 2011. http://www.cdc.gov/mmwr/preview/mmwrhtml/mm5114a2.html.

"Chapter 10 Vocal Registers," *Tutorial based on Ingo Titze's Principles of Voice Production* (Englewood Cliffs, NJ: Prentice Hall, 1994). The National Center for Voice and Speech. Accessed August 21, 2011. http://www.ncvs.org/ncvs/tutorials/voiceprod/tutorial/voluntary.html

Cone, Barbara, Patricia Dorn, Dawn Konrad-Martin, Jennifer Lister, Candice Ortiz, and Kim Schairer. "Ototoxic Medications (Medication Effects)." *American Speech-Language-Hearing Association.* Last modified 2011. Accessed January 27, 2011. http://www.asha.org/public/hearing/Ototoxic-Medications.

Dangerous Decibels. "Decibel Exposure Time Guidelines." Last modified 2011. Accessed January 27, 2011. http://www.dangerousdecibels.org/research/information-center/decibel-exposure-time-guidelines.

"Is It Really Decaf?" *Consumer Reports*, November 2007, 7. Accessed November 24, 2010. http://www.consumerreports.org/cro/food/beverages/coffee-tea/is -it-really decaffeinated-coffee-11–07/overview/decaf-coffee-ov.html.

The Mayo Clinic. "Aerobic Exercise: How to Warm up and Cool Down." Last updated March 20, 2009. http://www.mayoclinic.com/health/exercise/SM00067.

Milton J. Dance Jr. Head and Neck Center at Greater Baltimore Medical Center. "Tips for Professional Voice Users and Singers." Copyright 2010. Accessed January 16, 2011. http://www.gbmc.org/home_voicecenter.cfm?id=1561.

Academy of Nutrition and Dietetics (formerly American Dietetic Association). Sports Nutrition Care Manual, Client Education > Endurance Athletes > Meal Planning Tips and Food Lists. Last modified 2010. Accessed January 16, 2012. http://nutritioncaremanual.org/content.cfm?ncm_content_id=110785.

Oxford Advanced Learners Dictionary. http://www.oxfordadvancedlearnersdictionary.com.

Schindler, Joshua, and Yvette Leslie. "Arytenoid Dislocation." *emedicine* from *WebMD.* Last modified January 7, 2010. http://emedicine.medscape.com/article/866464-overview.

Stark, Paul. "Radiology of the Trachea." Edited by Nestor L. Muller. UpToDate. Last modified October 13, 2009. Accessed December 11, 2010. http://www.uptodate.com/patients/content/topic.do?topicKey=~5CfPy6YkRYbqVI.

Zeratsky, Katherine. "Caffeine: Is It Dehydrating or Not?" *Nutrition and Healthy Eating.* Last modified August 21, 2009. http://www.mayoclinic.com/health/caffeinated-drinks/AN01661.

DATE DUE

JAN 3 2014			
JAN 3 1 2014			